MW01194865

GASP

AIRWAY HEALTH

THE HIDDEN PATH TO WELLNESS

Dr Michael Gelb
Dr Howard Hindin

GASP

AIRWAY HEALTH

THE HIDDEN PATH TO WELLNESS

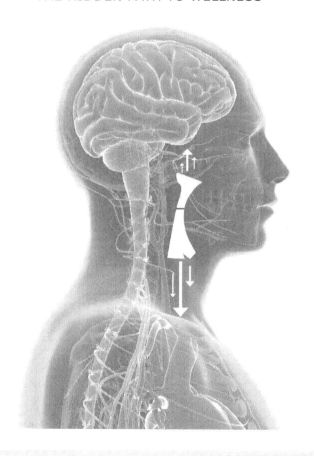

First Edition
Published by Dr Michael Gelb and Dr Howard Hindin
United States of America
For more information, visit:

www.GelbCenter.com and www.Hindincenter.com

Printed and bound in the USA

ISBN-10: 1536995266
ISBN-13: 978-1536995268

Layout and book design by www.abcmediasolutions.com
Editing by www.abcwriters.com

Dr Gelb: *I would like to dedicate this book to my parents Sally and Harold Gelb as well as my children Marissa and Clifford.*

Dr Hindin: *I am thankful for the many people who influenced and supported my journey of curiosity and learning that has led to the creation of GASP. Michael Gelb and I started with an idea, which grew into the writing team we created along with Carol Richardson. We constantly motivated each other with research we discovered, patient experiences we shared and the excitement of bringing the message of GASP to all that we know will benefit.*

GASP is dedicated to the many teachers who opened my eyes and mind to new ideas, to questions that did not make sense and to an understanding of the important role oral conditions play in health and disease. I stand on the shoulders of pioneers such as Harold Gelb, Myron Lieb, Willie May, Aelred Fonder, and Brendan Stack in tmj; Daniel Garliner in myofunctional therapy, John Witzig and Bill Hang in functional expansion orthodontics; and Carlton Fredericks, Michael Schachter, Ron Hoffman and Jeffrey Bland in nutrition. I am also grateful for the endless discussions that my good friend Peter Madill and I have been enjoying for over 30 years.

I am thankful and honored to practice with my son, Jeffrey Hindin, and his wife Jill Meyer-Hindin, who are doing their own pioneering work in the structure and function of the airway in the dental arena. And to my daughter Tami, (acupuncturist and cranial-sacral therapist), who continues to astonish me with wonderful results she achieves with infants, toddlers and children. Daily, I benefit from all my friends and colleagues in the airway/sleep world that share the passionate pursuit of discovery and knowledge. I am particularly thankful to my wife Rose, who is always there to listen and give support to the sometimes frustrating creative process.

GASP is dedicated to all the patients over the years that shared stories, successes and failures, and continually enforced the vital importance of the airway oral systemic connection. Finally, GASP is for all those who will be able to find understanding and hope for their own hidden airway problem.

CONTENTS

Part III- No Peak Performance Without the Breath of Life

Preface

Improper breathing and sleep patterns adversely affect health, mood, energy, focus and function, and if untreated will ultimately lead to multiple systemic disorders. We refer to this constellation of disorders as "hidden airway" problems since they so often go unrecognized. These problems express themselves in many ways, and typically the symptoms are treated but not the underlying problem. As a result, new expressions appear and they are treated with medications, surgery and other interventions. But the continued struggle for adequate breath leads to persistent inflammation and an assortment of chronic diseases. Non-restorative sleep leads to poor focus and function, as well as interruptions in growth, development and learning. Recently, even Alzheimer's disease, dementia and cancer have been linked to airway / sleep problems.

Narrow and constricted airways are a primary cause of systemic inflammation, oxidative stress and endothelial dysfunction. They are also a major contributing and perpetuating factor in cardiovascular disease, diabetes and refractory depression and anxiety.

The writing of *Gasp* came from a series of conversations that we—Howie Hindin and Michael Gelb—had concerning the overwhelming number of children and adults presenting with chronic pain, headaches, attention deficit hyperactivity disorder (ADHD), anxiety, depression and chronic fatigue. We shared our patient stories and successes—in particular, the miraculous changes we observed when patients' airway and sleep problems were recognized and properly diagnosed and treated. A large number of these patients came to our practices after seeing many, many other practitioners. One of us commented that we should never have to see these patients; their problems were present for years—maybe even from childhood. These problems were there to be treated earlier, or even prevented. That's right. We believe that snoring, sleep apnea and TMJ disorders can be prevented.

Michael: I grew up listening to my father—Dr Harold Gelb, a brilliant clinician, teacher and author—talk to his patients and other practitioners about the harmful effects of removing permanent adult premolar teeth prior to orthodontics, as well as the harmful effect of headgear. I came to understand early on that making the mouth smaller—either by filing down or removing healthy teeth or by orthodontically retracting healthy jaws—was detrimental to one's health. Unfortunately, most of the dental community strongly disagreed with these thoughts going back to the 1920s up until today. Even though the treatment results were compelling, a scientific explanation was lacking.

My mother, Sally, was a myofunctional therapist who worked with my father and I back in the 1980s. My father advocated a multidisciplinary approach working with many practitioners offering other modalities. Today we know that by intervening early with adenotonsilectomy, palatal expansion and Myofunctional therapy most cases of mouthbreathing, snoring and apnea can be successfully treated with long-lasting results. Think of the incredible public health benefits derived by investing in our children before age 5 in areas of brain development, and prevention of epigenetic changes.

Howard: I have been in practice for 50 years. My first connection to Michael was being introduced to the world of TMJ disorders and treatment by Harold Gelb in 1968. Our dental practice evolved to focus on the medical / dental connection working with many of the leading integrative practitioners. We would sometimes encounter remarkable health improvements when dental conditions like tooth infections, gum disease, and TMJ were uncovered and properly treated. Sometimes we were disappointed when we did not get the results we expected; something was missing. But when we added treatment for sleep, and then airway, our results improved. I remember listening to the radio reporter Paul Harvey tell stories with surprised endings and the line: "Now you know the rest of the story." In this case, the structure and function of the airway is the rest of the story.

The evidence we present in *Gasp* will change many of the paradigms in dentistry and medicine. We previously believed that by correcting TMJ pain and dysfunction, our patients were awakening better rested and more refreshed. We now know this: maintaining the jaws in a forward position at night maintains an open airway, which increases oxygenation and allows deeper stage 3 sleep and REM—restoring both body and mind. So it was serendipitously discovered, through overnight sleep studies and CBCT imaging, that keeping the lower jaw forward at night brings the tongue and soft palate forward and opens the airway.

Further evidence poured in from noted researchers like epidemiologist Karen Bonuck and physicians / researchers David Gozal and Christian Guilleminault. They found that mouthbreathing, snoring and sleep apnea can start at birth and lead to changes in the prefrontal cortex as early as the first year of life. The changes produced by snoring, apnea, flow limitation and resisted breathing in infants can therefore lead to executive function issues at age 4 and 7 with neurobehavioral and neurocognitive consequences. We knew that mouthbreathing could lead to altered growth patterns, which would exacerbate adult snoring and obstructive sleep apnea. This was a revelation because it helped Michael explain his own growth and development as well as some of his behavior patterns from childhood. It is now clear that the paradigm of diagnosis and treatment of these children needs to change. The crisis has reached epidemic proportions but these trends are reversible.

Integrative, functional and preventive medicine preaches health and wellness through diet, exercise, and a good mental attitude. Sometimes sleep is mentioned but not often or in the context of airway.

We have written *Gasp* to convey the stories of our patients and to share our experiences and what we have learned as dentists. We developed a new educational system called Airway Centric®. *Gasp* was written so anyone with children or parents or siblings can have hope, can uncover their hidden airway problem, and can find the help they need to be the best they can be—at any age. Dentists should play a key role on a *team* of healthcare practitioners working to establish a healthy airway at any age. Yes, it requires a team approach.

Gasp offers inspiration and hope. Current paradigms must change, and they are changing. We want to move the change along. We want this important information to reach those whose lives can be changed today. Early diagnosis and intervention is important. In at-risk children, treatment can start as early as 2.5 to 3 years of age. It is never too early or too late to intervene. We have seen patients, from 2 to 95 years old, benefit.

We also want to enlist each of you into our army for change. Read *Gasp*, and after you finish, you will begin to notice airway problems in the faces of family and friends—the mouth-breathers, the retracted jaws, the inattentive, sleepy child with slump shoulder and a forward head position—and more. Share this book and change a life; give it to your pediatrician and your pediatric dentist. There are pods of practitioners growing across the country trained in Airway Centric® dentistry and medicine.

This is our passion, so we have been instrumental in forming two groups:

1. The Foundation for Airway Health – to educate the public and increase awareness. (www.foundationforairwayhealth.org)

2. The American Academy of Physiological Medicine and Dentistry (AAPMD) – a place for all healthcare practitioners to learn and grow their knowledge of airway and functioning as part of a collaborative team. (www.AAPMD.org)

Introduction

This book is about inspiration and hope. We are drowning in a "tsunami of chronic disease" according to Dr Jeffrey Bland. This is a crisis of epic proportions. There have been huge increases in diabetes, dementia and other chronic diseases. And it is not only chronic disease; the number of children with ADHD has doubled, there is a 300% increase in obesity since 1980, and there are tremendous increases in those diagnosed with mental illness, anxiety, depression and more. These acquired diseases will cost our global economy more than $50 trillion over the next 20 years and will kill twice as many people as infectious diseases.

Are these staggering increases in ill health attributed to environmental factors? Are we paying the price, as Rachel Carson warned in *Silent Spring*, from the widespread use of pesticides following World War II? Is it diet and our sedentary lifestyle? Other causes might be microbes, allergens, toxins, and stress. The emerging field of Epigenetics helps explain how environmental changes can alter the expression of our genes in one lifetime and how much this expression has radically changed over the past 40 years.

Gasp looks at our healthcare crisis from a different angle. We are Homo sapiens, the most evolved species on earth. Evolution has blessed us by increasing the size of our brain, but this has led to small retracted faces and sinuses compared to our predecessors. As pollution has worsened and our diets have deteriorated, our jaws have narrowed and teeth are coming in crooked. There is rarely room for all 32 teeth these days. Our ability to speak was made possible by a flexible pharynx, but this created an "Achilles heel" of a collapsible airway. We are the only mammals except bulldogs who snore and stop breathing during sleep.

Gasp is about inspiration and hope. The word "inspiration" is related to the concepts of guidance, encouragement and motivation. Here is another meaning: the act of breathing or drawing a breath. *Gasp* is about all of this. It is about the "hidden airway" problem altering the lives of 50% of us. We call it "hidden" because it is often not looked for; it goes unrecognized and untreated. We offer the information in this book as a path to better airways and breathing, and to healthier and more energetic lives. We believe this book will be an inspiration for those who wrongly believe they were dealt a "bad hand" in life—that they must continue to suffer with an affliction that can be addressed.

This book is for the poor learners, those battling pain and fatigue and those who have been labeled "damaged, lacking will power and defective." It is for those individuals—of all ages—who are NOT defective but are struggling to breathe.

Gasp is about our airway, breathing and sleep. Problems can start at birth. Many premature babies are mouth breathers. A poorly structured and functioning airway leads to mouthbreathing, snoring and sleep apnea; it can interfere with restorative sleep and ultimately damage the part of the brain called the prefrontal cortex, which controls executive function skills, attentiveness, anxiety and depression. The information in this book will describe how to restore an ideal airway with early intervention and where to go for help. As these hidden airway problems are exposed, the paradigm of Ear, Nose and Throat doctors, allergists, pediatricians, orthodontists and dentists will evolve to encourage better recognition and diagnosis of airway-centered disorders as early as the first year of life. The reader will learn how once the airway is established with breastfeeding, allergy treatment, adenotonsillectomy and palatal expansion, then neurocognitive and neurobehavioral problems are greatly improved—often without any medication. Anxiety and depression are alleviated, and the behavior and performance of our kids are remarkably transformed.

Gasp is not only about the airway of our children. 50% of us have a life limited by an airway or a sleep disorder.

Today there is a health movement toward "Wellness." Wellness is about diet and nutrition, exercise, and mental attitude. The new paradigm popularized by Mark Hyman, Jeffrey Bland and Drs Amen and Perlmutter is called "Functional Medicine." It addresses the causes of chronic disease with an individualized approach and emphasizes early intervention. It restores the balance amongst functional systems and the networks that connect them.

What is the missing link? It is *airway, breathing* and *sleep.* Breathing is life. If we don't breathe we die. If we don't breathe well when we sleep, 1/3 of our life is affected. If you work harder to breathe during the day, everything you do will be more difficult or even impossible. Gasp tells you why and how this works.

Gasp describes the impact of a narrowed airway from cradle to grave. Every day, we encounter fatigued patients with chronic headaches and neck pain. They have difficulty concentrating; they suffer with GI problems from acid reflux to irritable bowel syndrome. They range from thin women to men who have put on a few pounds. And you do not have to be obese to have an airway problem. Many of our younger patients with ADHD and airway issues have little body fat.

How important is an open airway? Time after time we see that once the airway is opened during the day and maintained during sleep, the transformation is quick and dramatic. You will read about how Valerie Deegan found her son Connor Deegan. He went from wishing he was dead, temper tantrums and D's and F's to his delightful former self getting A's and B's again.

Adults get their mojo back. They sleep through the night and awaken refreshed. Their lives are extended but more importantly they feel better and have less systemic inflammation. Eyes open up and brighten and skin tone glows. *Why?* Our patients suffer from intermittent hypoxia or oxygen desaturations as well as sleep fragmentation or disturbed sleep. This produces widespread systemic inflammation, oxidative stress and endothelial dysfunction, which affects the blood vessels and cardiovascular system. Cardiovascular and cerebrovascular diseases are highly correlated with obstructive sleep apnea as is refractory depression.

We are continually amazed to see how insomnia and anxiety improve once we open the airway and allow for easier breathing. It's as if we are removing hands that were strangling the neck. The threat is removed, breathing is easier and anxiety and insomnia improve.

Recent studies demonstrate that the seeds of dementia and Alzheimer's disease may be planted decades earlier with chronic airway and sleep disorders. It may take years to establish enough scientific proof. Do you want to consciously make the choice to wait? Managing the airway and obstructive sleep apnea with CPAP and oral appliance therapy or weight loss may possibly reduce the risk of—or even prevent entirely—these diseases, and these approaches will certainly lead to more optimal health, function and happiness. It is so important to begin treatment as early as possible, starting with snoring in adults and mouthbreathing in children.

Airway Centric® dentistry places the airway above all else. The hierarchy for dentists should be airway first then TMJ and clenching or bruxism, and lastly the teeth, bite and occlusion. Sleep specialists like Christian Guilleminault from Stanford University agree that airway-centered disorders can be prevented by intervention in early childhood. We now know through the study of epigenetics that we need not suffer the fate of our parents' genes. We can change the expression of our genes through nutrigenomics and by incorporating supplements, diet, reading to our children, pollution free environment and Airway Centric® medicine.

Facial structures can be optimized if they are constructed around an open, well-functioning airway. This requires collaboration between pediatrician, ENT, allergist, pediatric dentist, orthodontist, speech language pathologist and myofunctional therapist. Gasp will help find and build the "airway team" for you.

The time for *Gasp* is now! Doing nothing is not an option. An Airway Centric® approach to wellness and lifestyle is simple and easy at any age, from birth through old age.

Breathe and be inspired!

Part I - It's All About Airways

1

C H A P T E R

Gasping for Life?

Are you constantly grappling with health problems such as fatigue, excess weight, headaches, chronic pain, sugar and junk food cravings, or with stress in general?

Do you have a child with learning disabilities, ADHD, behavioral issues, chronic ear and nose infections, allergies, or asthma?

Is your doctor treating you or your child for a chronic disease like high blood pressure, diabetes, obesity, insomnia, thyroid or autoimmune disorders, anxiety, or depression?

What if you discovered that there is one potential cause underlying all of these conditions?

Of course, many factors can lead to these problems, but one factor is rarely considered by today's medical practitioners, and the time has come for a change. This silent health saboteur should be top-of-mind for the millions of Americans—adults, parents, and young people alike—who suffer from these and other related chronic illnesses. The research and clinical stories in this book will shed light on this underlying cause of so many health and learning issues, and we hope it will ultimately become a primary consideration of every healthcare practitioner, from pediatricians to cardiologists.

We're talking about airway-centered disorder, or ACD.

ACD is a physiological disorder of the mouth, jaw, nasal passages, tongue, or throat that involves an obstruction of the upper airways and in turn leads to breathing difficulties, including mouth breathing, snoring, sleep apnea, hypopneas, and upper airway resistance syndrome (UARS). These disorders can be precursors to a variety of more complex and pervasive health, developmental, and behavioral issues.

Sleep-Disordered Breathing (SDB) symptoms:

» Headaches
» Snoring
» Difficulty sleeping
» Neck, jaw, or ear pain
» Sugar cravings
» Junk food cravings
» Obesity
» Type 2 Diabetes
» Cardiovascular Disease
» Difficulty focusing mentally
» Excessive Daytime sleepiness
» Low energy
» Wake up feeling unrefreshed

ACD leads to either partial or complete blockages of the nasal passages or throat, which can affect breathing 24 hours a day. Research has extensively documented the negative effects of breathing difficulties during sleep, so we will focus primarily on these issues, collectively known as sleep-disordered breathing, or SDB.

These terms may be unfamiliar to you (and perhaps even to your doctor), but you'll become acquainted with them in the coming chapters. For now, it's important to know that ACD—which can begin at birth—affects how we breathe because it increases the amount of effort we put into breathing just to survive. People with ACD find it difficult to thrive and often experience significant health issues, as illustrated by the many stories in this book.

Deep, restorative sleep is essential to survival, as well as to our ability to thrive at all ages and stages of life. ACD causes disrupted or fragmented sleep with profoundly disturbing effects on the brain. It causes systemic inflammation, oxidative stress, and a host of severe health problems, like impaired functioning of the arteries (endothelial dysfunction).

ACD can lead to learning and behavior disorders such as attention deficit hyperactivity disorder (ADHD). It is also a causative factor in obesity, allergies, asthma, diabetes, heart disease, stroke, depression, anxiety, erectile dysfunction, and Alzheimer's disease. Because ACD prevents deeply restorative sleep, it can affect—or even destroy—relationships and work performance. In addition to physical impairment, ACD impairs your ability to function intelligently and stay focused. Moreover, the brain often reacts to ACD during sleep by inducing a physiological response, which may involve any or all of the following: a craving for sugary foods, hyperactivity, anxiety, or irritability. These tendencies exacerbate the health problems we've already mentioned.

If that sounds like a huge chunk to bite off, it is!

If you're saying to yourself, "I've never heard of this," you're not alone. Although your doctor may be aware of sleep-disordered breathing, he or she likely has never considered its prevalence and all the ramifications.

In this book, you will learn about ACD; how to recognize it in yourself, your children, and other members of your family; and where to go for care. We've written this book to help you take charge of your own health and your family's health. You'll discover all the signs of ACD and SDBs (sleep-disordered breathing disorders), and since you will be equipped to recognize them, you'll also know how to find the medical allies you need to resolve the problem.

Ideal health, wellness, and brain development are dependent upon an open airway, nasal breathing, and deep, restorative sleep. Recent medical studies show us exactly why this is true. Yet somehow, this basic concept has all-too-frequently escaped the attention of today's medical professionals.

As human beings, we will do anything and everything to breathe, because breathing is our most important life-giving function. To breathe, we must have an open airway. Healthcare providers can either *improve* our ability to breathe or *worsen* it. In fact, those of us who specialize in airway health and dentistry have come to understand ourselves primarily as health care practitioners—and also as primary care givers who can help save your life.

We have over 70 years of combined experience in dentistry and preventive health care. We understand that opening your airway (not surgically, of course, but using nighttime appliances, orthodontia and other treatment modalities) can have a dramatic impact on your ability to function in everyday life, on your physical appearance, and on your general health. Our number one responsibility as dentists—and healthcare practitioners—is to help you breathe by providing an open airway. Dentists can suggest various treatments to open airways in people of all ages, and we will explain these treatment options in this book.

"You know we have an epidemic of Obstructive Sleep Apnea when you see a 'travel CPAP' machine for sale in the Sky Mall magazine" (while flying across the United States)." – Kaitlyn Tarbert, RDH, a Pediatric Oral Myofunctional Therapist

This new, interdisciplinary approach to dentistry as healthcare—called the Airway Centric® Model—aims at preventing airway-centered disorders, sleep-disordered breathing, and all the associated challenges to mental and physical health. The Airway Centric® Model of diagnosis and treatment enables people of all ages to sleep and breathe more effectively so they can function better in all areas of life. The Airway Centric® Model trumps anything in dentistry and perhaps even in all of healthcare, because breathing is essential to life.

We've all been told that diet, exercise, and a good night's sleep are the keys to handling life's stressors. But being able to take a deep breath is equally important. There are many reasons why breathing effectively has become more challenging for many people, especially during sleep. Most of these challenges relate to airway dysfunction. Airway dysfunction is one of many precursors to diseases that cause lifelong suffering, and it is too often overlooked. We point to it not only to raise awareness among medical practitioners across a variety of specialties, but more importantly to raise awareness among parents who can help prevent life-long suffering in their children, as well as among all adults suffering from chronic health problems that may be influenced by sleep-disordered breathing.

We believe airway-centered disorders, in their various forms, are a missing link in medicine today. In fact, we know that in most cases, our Airway Centric® approach provides relief from symptoms and prompts a return to health.

In simple terms, this program is a way of life. It is a paradigm shift that puts proper breathing, open airways, and restful sleep at the center of prevention and treatment plans—rather than at the far edge of a doctor's radar screen, where it has remained for too long. ACD and sleep-disordered breathing are preventable and treatable at any age.

We offer this book as a beacon of hope for those who are frustrated by any of a number of health challenges that have confounded modern medicine for too long. We believe you'll find the answers to your problems here.

2

C H A P T E R

What Happened to Our Airways?

Face Forward

Fifty years ago, Marilyn Monroe's iconic beauty graced the big screen. Even now, more than 50 years after her death, she is still an icon of beauty and sensuality. Her prominent cheekbones, straight nose, and full lips represent the ideal of femininity. Notice her wide jawline with its strong chin and that beautifully broad smile. Monroe's beauty features also happen to be signs of a healthy airway.

A generation later, the Oscar-winning actor Robert Redford epitomized the rugged blond handsomeness and all-American athleticism that made him the heartthrob of millions of women. His strong jaw line and broad face evoke masculine strength. They are also a sign of a healthy airway.

Instinctively, we see a healthy face as a beautiful one. In other words, "gorgeous" faces are nature's way of leading us to healthy mates, who offer the best chances of creating healthy and beautiful offspring. Human beings are hard-wired to respond sexually to healthy partners. Call it natural selection, but after all, the goal of sexuality is procreation and the preservation of our own individual gene pool and the human race. Furthermore, throughout life in many societies, attractive people tend to have advantages, as though our instinct is to pay attention to and to trust people who are healthy.

Although beauty is definitely in the eye of the beholder, and the personification of it comes in many different shapes and sizes, most people tend to agree on a starting point for defining beauty: prominent cheeks, full lips, straight teeth, a wide strong jawline, and a mouth without an overbite or receded jaw.

You can probably guess where we are going here: It is no co-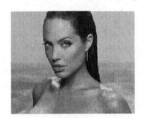incidence that these standards of beauty are also indications that the airway is open and clear. But in the generations between Monroe and Redford's heyday and today's Hollywood stars, faces have changed.

Consider Angelina Jolie. Certainly she's gorgeous. But her face is much narrower than Monroe's and there are rumors that she has had plastic surgery: rhinoplasty to straighten and thin her nose, implants to strengthen her chin, and silicone injections to enhance her pouty lips.

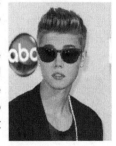

Why would anyone do that? Because the effect calls to mind the bloom of youth and good health, and healthy is beautiful. But does it change what is underneath—the airway? It is possible to change the structures underneath, but this is not what plastic surgeons are trained to do.

Now let's consider Justin Bieber, the current young generation's heartthrob. Though Bieber makes the preteen crowd swoon, his long narrow face, pug nose, tiny mouth and open lips are a far cry from the rugged masculinity of Robert Redford.

Bieber represents a generation of children who were less often breastfed and who were weaned to soft diets—baby cereals and pureed foods, and then sugary cereals designed to appeal to children, hot dogs, luncheon meats, and other soft foods which have become prominent in the "standard American diet."[1] (We'll get into more about why and how a soft diet affects face structure in a bit.) They also come from the first generation raised in a highly toxic environment.

It's interesting to note that both Bieber and Jolie have their mouths partly open. Perhaps they think this is sexy. We have to ask, though: are they simply mouth-breathers? And is this the new "normal"?

It's clear: In today's Western world, jaws are narrower and pushed back, noses are pushed in, and faces are longer and narrower—all typical results from a lack of breastfeeding, soft diets, and mouth breathing that have become commonplace. If you find this argument hard to swallow, read on; we will connect the scientific dots for you.

These facial characteristics coincide with a rounded, forward shoulder posture as well as a forward head posture. A jaw that does not develop forward during childhood will often continue to recede throughout life, leading to that characteristic "hump" or bump in the middle of the nose as the recession pulls the tip of the nose downward. All of these less-than-ideal features are telltale signs of blocked airways.

Interestingly, an attractive face and an open airway go hand in hand. A healthy face grows proportionally, as well as balanced in both the forward direction and horizontally. In fact, a healthy face is not only gorgeous when viewed straight on, but the profile is attractive as well, with the forehead and chin in the same plumb line. For that type of face to develop, a person's airway must be open and functioning from birth through adulthood.

A Little Bit of History

Let's go back over 12,000 years to a time before the development of agriculture, when our ancestors lived in nature, hunting and gathering their food. Our skulls and faces were much more ape-like,

---

1 It is not by coincidence that this term was coined as the acronym "SAD," because the standard American diet is sadly lacking in nutritional quality.

with wide jaws and rounded facial structures. About 12,000 years ago, humanity developed agriculture, and along with a settled agrarian lifestyle, human beings began to eat a "softer" diet.

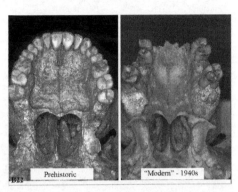

Figure 1. Source: http://www.brianpalmerdds.com/pdf/adsm_section_b.pdf
used with permission of Dr Kevin Boyd, DDS, MS

As you can see in Figure 1, ancient skulls had a wide, rounded arch on the upper jaw, along with large, wide nasal openings to the sinuses, creating nicely open airways through the sinuses. Because the lower jaw was also wide and rounded, there was plenty of room for the tongue, and the jaw could comfortably rest in a forward position, creating open airways in the throat as well. By contrast, the 1940s skull has a narrow, V-shaped arch, small nasal passages, and not much room for the tongue (along with a lot of evident tooth decay).

The staples of a hunter-gatherer lifestyle, up until that era, were meat, fruit, and nuts (effectively, the Paleo diet) along with wild grains and vegetables. Most of this diet was uncooked and difficult to chew. The softer diet introduced with agriculture 10,000 years ago contained more vegetables and grains, which were typically cooked, along with fruits and cooked meats (cooking makes meat softer).

According to researchers such as Boyd and Harvard evolutionary biologist Daniel Lieberman, this soft diet eliminated the natural need for chewing, and this began to change the shapes of our faces: narrowing our jaws and creating restrictions in our airways. Lieberman performed a study on pigs, feeding one group a soft diet and one group foods that were tough to chew. The group that ate tough food developed not only stronger muscles but also larger jaws, while the group with soft foods developed weaker, smaller jaws. It took only one generation to create these smaller jaws. The theory is that this is what happened to human beings; rather than a *genetic* change in the short span of 10,000 years, an *epigenetic effect* has occurred because of soft diets, resulting in smaller faces and narrower jaws.[2]

In fact, the research of Dr Robert Corruccini of Southern Illinois University shows just this result. Dr Corruccini studied populations that had not yet been affected by Western cultures as they became westernized and began to eat the soft, sugary foods of Western industrialized cultures.

Corruccini found that there was virtually no malocclusion (bad bite due to poor development of the jaws) in these cultures *before* Western diets were introduced. Within one generation of the introduction of the Western diet, 50% of the population developed malocclusion. Within two generations, 70% of the population had malocclusion. The third generation eating an industrialized diet had 85% malocclusion. This poor formation of the jaws is an epidemic of industrialized cultures today.[3]

Smaller jaws leave less room for teeth, causing crowding. They also leave less room for the tongue, forcing it to move backwards, especially during sleep, where it tends to block the airway. With

---

2 See Kevin Boyd, M.Sc., DDS, "Darwinian Dentistry, Part 1: An Evolutionary Perspective on the Etiology of Malocclusion," *JAOS* November/December 2011, pp. 34-40, available on: www.orthodontics.com, and Jonathan Shaw, "Head to Toe: Daniel Lieberman tracks the evolution of the human head," *Harvard Magazine*, January/February 2011, pp. 25-29.

3 See: R.S. Corruccini. 1984. An Epidemiologic Transition in Dental Occlusion in World Populations. *American Journal of Orthodontics* 86 (5): 419-426, also *How Anthropology Informs the Orthodontic Diagnosis of Malocclusion's Causes*, Lewiston: Edwin Mellen Press, 1999, and http://wholehealthsource.blogspot.com/2009/09/malocclusion-disease-of-civilization.html. This information was obtained during a lecture by Dr Ben Miraglia, DDS, Airway Centric® Orthodontist during a lecture on March 27, 2014 in Hartsdale NY, hosted by the AAPMD.

smaller faces and narrower jaws have also come smaller nasal openings in the back of the mouth (above the palate). (See figure 1)

In the last 200 years, since the beginning of the Industrial Revolution, and particularly in the last 35 years, our faces generally have flattened and narrowed even more. We're slowly developing "bulldog-like" faces as our noses and sinuses are increasingly pushed in, making nasal breathing difficult and causing ACD.

Several factors have contributed to this narrowing of our airways. Dentist and researcher Kevin Boyd coined the term "Darwinian Dentistry" to refer to the perspective of normative and healthy aspects in the human jaw and mouth, based on studies of human skulls from different time periods and cultures. This field of study is also called Evolutionary Oral Medicine, and it's an important de-velopment in our efforts to understand why so many people have developed narrow airways.[4]

Here's how breastfeeding—or not—relates to airway problems. As women left home to work during the Industrial Revolution, there was less and less breastfeeding. Breastfeeding of infants is a primary factor in normal facial development because the newborn's sucking action (which is not replicated in bottle-feeding) develops muscles critical to proper airway development. In addition, as Boyd points out, it was during the development of the Industrial Revolution that infant formulas and "convenience foods" such as soft baby cereals were commercially developed.[5]

As more and more women worked outside the home, particu-larly from the 1980s on, breastfeeding continued to fall out of favor, and also the demand for fast foods and convenience foods rapidly expanded. Diets therefore changed radically; in particular they included more soft foods. Our food also became more processed and chemically laden.

The result of these dietary changes has been smaller jaws, just as Harvard evolutionary biologist Daniel Lieberman found in his

---

4 Boyd, "Darwinian Dentistry, Part 1"

5 Boyd, Kevin, "Darwinian Dentistry, Part 2: Early Childhood Nutrition, Dentofacial Development and Chronic Disease," *JAOS* March/April 2012, pp. 28-32.

study with pigs.[6] These post-Industrial Revolution dietary changes translate directly to humans who "never have to actually chew anything all day long," says Lieberman,[7] resulting in narrower faces and small jaws with insufficient room for teeth. Not only that, noses, sinuses and breathing passages are markedly smaller today than they were just a generation ago.

How can we understand the impact of these external factors on our internal facial structures? It all goes to a new science called epigenetics that links environmental factors to phenotypic expression of our genes.[8] One link, as shown in some studies of the jaw, is through the development of the musculature, which actually shapes bone formation during development. As a baby breastfeeds, the nipple repeatedly presses against the palate as the milk is expressed. This pressure widens and expands the palate as it develops. In addition, a baby's muscles have to work hard to pump the milk; this action pulls on the jaw and bony sutures of the mouth in such a way that more bone is deposited and the jaws are widened.[9] By contrast, bottle-feeding and sucking on pacifiers does not contribute to the widening of the jaws, but instead causes higher palates and narrower jaws.[10]

Humans are the only mammal in which the epiglottis descends between six months and one year of age, leaving the airway susceptible behind the tongue and soft palate. During breastfeeding the epiglottis is locked with the soft palate, allowing the channeling of milk into the stomach.

Humans are the only mammal with a free floating hyoid bone, which also makes the airway vulnerable. All other mammals have a strutted hyoid, which protects airway integrity.

Because of our upright posture, the airway in humans has a 90 degree turn, which creates turbulence while breathing, compared to four-legged mammals which have a much straighter and therefore

---

6 Jonathan Shaw, "Head to Toe: Daniel Lieberman tracks the evolution of the human head," *Harvard Magazine*, January/February 2011, p. 27.

7 Ibid.

8 See, for instance, http://www.sciencemag.org/content/330/6004/611

9 See Boyd, "Darwinian Dentistry, Part 2," p. 30.

10 Ibid.

more open airway. As the brain of *Homo sapiens* enlarged, the jaws and sinuses were pushed back as our faces flattened and shrunk.

All this is to say that our human physiology sets us up to be vulnerable to airway blockages. With changes in our diets and a lack of breastfeeding, the natural mechanisms for creating healthy jaws and airways have been inhibited. On top of that, we have added thousands of industrial chemicals into our environment in the last five decades. These chemicals have infiltrated our air and our water, our homes, our food, and our personal care products.

We became painfully aware of the ravages of pesticides on our inner and outer environments after Rachel Carson published her iconic book, *Silent Spring* in 1962. Since then, the picture worsened. A 2009 Environmental Working Group report showed 232 toxic chemicals in the cord blood of babies born in 2004, including mercury, fire retardants, pesticides, and Teflon chemicals.[11] This means that even unborn babies cannot escape exposure to chemical pollution.

We are now exposed to these pesticides and other toxic substances on a daily basis. This may be a primary factor in the profound changes in human physiology that have occurred in a startlingly short period of time. Scientists are just beginning to discover the variety of epigenetic changes that have resulted from these substances.

One of the most researched issues of exposure to pesticides and dioxins is the increased prevalence of cleft palates in children.[12] Exposure to toxic substances in the environment has been linked to lower IQs and learning disabilities in children.[13] Finally among these epigenetic effects, we also know that pollution causes increases in asthma and allergies. Allergies in turn lead to sleep-disordered breathing in both children and adults.[14] In other words, pollution

---

11 http://www.ewg.org/research/minority-cord-blood-report/bpa-and-other-cord-blood-pollutants

12 See, for instance: http://www.ncbi.nlm.nih.gov/pubmed/17608552 and http://hmg.oxfordjournals.org/content/8/10/1853.full

13 http://www.thelancet.com/journals/lancet/article/PIIS0140-6736(06)69665-7/fulltext

14 See, for instance, this study of 20,000 school-aged children in China: http://respiratory-research.com/content/11/1/144/abstract "Habitual

contributes to the epidemic of airway obstruction and sleep-disordered breathing.

The Perfect Storm

The result of all these epigenetic effects of our modern lifestyles is a perfect storm for our children's health involving: allergies, sinusitis, mouth breathing, snoring, sleep apnea and other forms of sleep-disordered breathing. Dr William M. Hang, DDS, MSD calls to our attention the crisis of airway development:

> "Few children in industrialized societies eating the Western diet and breathing pollutants have adequate immune systems allowing them to combat the allergens well enough to maintain nasal breathing, maintain proper oral posture and, therefore, ideal facial growth."[15]

It can hardly be coincidental that since the early 1980s— when our epigenetic exposures increased exponentially—obesity, diabetes, and cardiovascular disease rates have increased alarmingly, as have behavioral and learning disorders like ADHD. If you think that sounds like the consequences of ACD, as we mentioned in chapter one, you are absolutely right. We believe that all of these challenges to human health are intertwined, and that the one primary factor we can address is our airways.

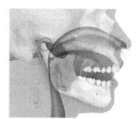

Figure 1: Blocked Airway

According to Lieberman, even long ago, as our brains became bigger, our faces flattened, and our jaws were pushed back (retruded). Unknowingly, and with good intentions, conventional dentistry and orthodontics have contributed to a worsening of this trend, because when teeth are pulled, the jaw becomes smaller. Even removing wisdom teeth can contribute to a smaller jaw. A smaller jaw means a smaller airway. The placing of headgear to

Snoring in school-aged children: environmental and biological predictors" Shenghui Li, Xinming Jin, Chonghuai Yan, Shenghu Wu, Fan Jiang and Xiaoming Shen. Also see: http://www.sleepreviewmag.com/2010/09/pollution-temperature-related-to-sleep-disordered-breathing/

15 https://www.facefocused.com/obstructive-sleep-apnea.html

pull the lower jaw back to correct malocclusion also compromises the airway. (See Figure 1)

As a result, airway-centered disorders are now very common in all ages across the United States. According to the National Institutes of Health, "obstructive sleep apnea (OSA) affects approximately 20% of US adults, of whom about 90% are undiagnosed."[16]

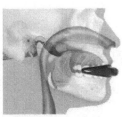

Data from the US Public Health Service's National Health and Nutrition Examination Survey, 2005-2006, show that 53.7% of men snore three or more nights per week; 14.5% of men snort, gasp, or stop breathing three or more nights per week; and 6.1% of men have been diagnosed with sleep apnea.[17] Assuming that the 6.1% who have been diagnosed with sleep apnea may be included in the other two numbers, that's approximately 70% of men who report having some form of sleep-disordered breathing!

Figure 2: Open Airway

For women, the total is approximately 40%, but that does not include the potential presence of UARS, a milder form of upper airway resistance during sleep that tends to happen in women and that is not yet broadly recognized (even among sleep study centers), and which therefore remains mostly undiagnosed. In fact, some studies show that up to 93% of women and 82% of men with signs and symptoms of moderate to severe forms of SDB are undiagnosed.[18]

Dr John Remmers, the Harvard-trained physician who coined the term Obstructive Sleep Apnea, states that OSA is becoming the most common chronic disease in industrialized countries.[19]

---

16 Finkel, KJ, et al, "Prevalence of Undiagnosed Obstructive Sleep Apnea among Adult Surgical Patients in an Academic Medical Center," *Sleep*, 2009, Aug; 10(7):753-8. http://www.ncbi.nlm.nih.gov/pubmed/19186102

17 http://www.thoracic.org/education/breathing-in-america/resources/chapter-23-sleep-disordered-breathing.pdf

18 http://www.thoracic.org/education/breathing-in-america/resources/chapter-23-sleep-disordered-breathing.pdf

19 https://www.facefocused.com/obstructive-sleep-apnea.html

The time has come for an Airway Centric® approach to dentistry and orthodontics, so that we widen jaws and open airways. (See Figure 2.) Our ability to breathe, sleep, stay healthy, and function at our best in life depends on an open airway.

3

C H A P T E R

The Airway Centric® Solution

O ur modern lifestyle has caused an epidemic of airway-centered disorders that have had disastrous effects on our national health. The toll has been terrible.

More and more children are being diagnosed with ADHD (attention deficit hyperactivity disorder). Between 1980 and 2007, there was an almost 700% increase of ADHD in the United States.[1] Granted, some of this increase may simply suggest greater awareness of the disorder among diagnosing professionals, along with possible misdiagnoses. Nevertheless, in the 1970s, less than 1% of American school children had ADHD. In the 1980s, the prevalence rose to 3-5%, and by 2011/12, the National Survey on Children's Health reported that 7.9% of all children ages 2 to 17 had ADHD and 7.6% were using medications for ADHD, emotions,

1 As reported by Sanford C. Newmark, M.D., of the UCSF Osher Center for Integrative Medicine, Pediatric Integrative Neurodevelopmental Clinic, on this site: http://www.parentseducationnetwork.org/Resources/Documents/PENHandout_Newmark030113.pdf

concentration, or behavior.[2] Increasing numbers of children have learning disabilities. As of 2004-2005, more than 13% of all children were enrolled in programs for learning disabilities.[3]

Now let's look at obesity statistics.

Childhood obesity has more than doubled since 1980, and adolescent obesity has quadrupled, according to the Centers for Disease Control and Prevention (CDC).[4] Today, nearly one-third of all children under 18 are overweight or obese, a startling increase of nearly 500%.[5]

Adult obesity trends in the same time period are equally shocking: 69.2% of all American adults are overweight or obese according to the National Institutes of Health.[6] Between 1980 and 2008 (the latest year for which figures are available), the obesity rate among adults in the United States doubled and the World Health Organization reports overweight and obesity have doubled worldwide since 1980.[7]

Clearly, ADHD and obesity have reached epidemic proportions. The question you may be asking is: How do ADHD and obesity relate to airway-centered disorder (ACD)?

The ability to breathe properly and deeply is vitally connected to deep and restorative sleep. Recent research shows that deep, uninterrupted sleep of adequate duration is necessary to keep our bodies healthy. Moreover, breathing properly during sleep is intimately tied to maintaining healthy brain chemistry.

Inadequate breathing (SDBs) cause a variety of sleep disorders ranging from mouth breathing and snoring to obstructive sleep apnea, hypopneas and upper airway resistance syndrome (UARS), a form that more commonly affects women. Research strongly links these sleep related breathing disorders with behavioral and

---

2 http://www.childhealthdata.org/browse/survey/results?q=2487&r=1

3 http://futureofchildren.org/publications/journals/article/index.xml?journalid=77&articleid=562&sectionid=3889

4 http://www.cdc.gov/healthyyouth/obesity/facts.htm

5 http://www.eatingdisorderpro.com/2012/04/16/childhood-obesity-a-norton-center-infographic/

6 http://win.niddk.nih.gov/statistics/

7 http://www.who.int/gho/ncd/risk_factors/obesity_text/en/

learning disabilities, emotional and psychological health, as well as obesity, diabetes, and cardiovascular disease.

This is a national crisis. Research has documented the link between ACD and SDBs with ADHD, anxiety, obesity, and other health problems. Our hope is that this information will spur physicians, dentists, and other health care providers to re-double the effort to include open airways as a critical part of all health programs.

Conventional attempts to address these health issues aren't working. The increased cost of managing the thousands of people with chronic illnesses has stressed our healthcare system and is bankrupting families and contributing to fiscal crisis in our country.

> An open and functioning airway is the top priority in the well-being of the human organism

Why is this all happening? Are we missing something?

Sure, doctors recognize the mounting rates of chronic diseases and disorders. But do they know why? Unfortunately, training leads most Western physicians to focus on treatment of *symptoms* rather than on *underlying causes* and *prevention*, so most of modern medicine has not yet considered sleep-disordered breathing and its effects on the body and brain.

The Airway Centric® Approach

As dentists, we have observed the consequences of airway problems for years. We have observed numerous—and seemingly un-resolvable—health issues in children and adults, health issues with roots in poor sleep quality, which in turn was due to sleep-disordered breathing. Once this problem is addressed, many of our patients achieve dramatic resolution of their chronic pain and other health issues.

We're a small but growing corps of believers. The time has come for physicians and health professionals in all fields to become aware of ACD as an underlying cause of these epidemic health and learning issues. Treating ACD can lead to a healthier future for Americans of all ages. After all, if there is no breath, there is no life. Fortunately, the great news is that these airway-related issues are preventable and treatable. While early treatment is always best (we have even treated newborns), ACD can be improved—and often even reversed—at any stage in life.

All it takes is recognition of the problem.

What is Airway Centric®?

Airway Centric® is a revolutionary system aimed at recognizing and correcting ACD. The first step is *observation*, because 27% of our children may have some form of abnormal breathing and abnormal facial anatomy, and this largely remains unrecognized by both parents and health care providers.[8]

We start by observing pregnant mothers, then children at birth, to recognize the signs and symptoms of sleep-disordered breathing. Parents are the first caretakers who need to observe their child with sensitivity to airway function, followed by obstetricians, pediatricians, lactation consultants, doulas, midwives, pediatric ENTs (ear, nose and throat specialists), pediatric sleep specialists, myofunctional therapists, oral surgeons, pediatric dentists and orthodontists.

The Airway Centric® approach calls upon these health care providers to focus on the role of the airway in disease prevention. Moreover, the Airway Centric® approach solicits a broader, more integrative approach to medicine. This Airway Centric® philosophy necessitates a paradigm shift in the medical community. Modern medicine has made great strides

Airway Centric®:

» A new approach to health based on prioritizing our ability to breathe well, especially during sleep.

» Emphasizes prevention and treatment

» Starts with parents observing their children while they sleep from birth onwards

» Includes physicians and healthcare providers

» Allows dentists and orthodontists to become part of a collaborative team of caregivers

---

8 See Gozal, David, "Obstructive Sleep Apnea in Children: Implications for the Developing Central Nervous System," http://www.ncbi.nlm.nih.gov/pmc/articles/PMC2490595/

with more specialized care, new procedures and ever increasing numbers of new and improved medications. But this specialization and narrowing of focus has had its drawbacks.

Modern medicine operates like the blind men who encountered an elephant in Aesop's fable. Each one focused on one detail from his experience. One man took hold of the trunk and said elephants must be like snakes, another held the tusk and said elephants were sharp like spears and yet another held the ear, saying elephants are thin and flexible, and so on. Of course, an elephant is all of those things, and so much more. Yet, no one sees the full picture and how everything fits as part of the whole.

Our medical system of specialists operates in much the same fashion. A cardiologist treats high blood pressure and does the surgeries for stents, bypasses and ablations. Psychiatrists treat people with depression, anxiety and ADHD. An internist may treat fatigue or digestive issues. Neurologists treat headaches and back pain. Urologists treat erectile dysfunction.

> Modern Medicine is approached like The Five Blind Men and the Elephant:
> One feels the trunk, one the tail, one the tusk, one the leg, and one the ear, but no one sees The Whole Elephant.

When specialists talk to each other, they are usually missing a critical piece. Like the blind men and the elephant, rarely do they put the pieces of the "elephant" together to see the larger picture of a patient's health problems. We health-care consumers, as parents or patients, must educate ourselves and hire medical practitioners who are able to see the "big picture" view of the patient.

The goal of the Airway Centric® approach is to do precisely that: show the big picture of health at all ages and stages of life, with open airways standing as the central basis of all health and well-being. In fact, each of the conditions treated by the specialists mentioned above may entail a blocked airway as a risk factor for the patients being treated.

Yet, airway impairment might not be recognized at all by the specialists examining the "elephant": there are many healthcare professionals who might see indications of airway obstructions early in life, and yet not recognize it for what it is. The obstetrician will deliver a premature infant. The lactation counselor could observe poor breastfeeding or a tight tongue attachment. The pediatrician checks for ear infections, allergies and developmental problems. The pediatric ENT might evaluate enlarged tonsils and adenoids or put tubes in the ears. The pediatric dentist might note that a child has an open-lipped posture and slack muscles around the mouth, jaws and face; or the preschool teacher might see the sleepy yet hyperactive child. All of these conditions indicate the potential presence or development of ACD.

The Team Approach

Early observation and treatment helps, but someone has to be in place to connect the dots and see the whole "elephant" for the large and pervasive problem it is. Part of a parent's role is to become fearless in advocating for their children.

We encourage a thorough evaluation of children's airways, and after diagnosis, a program of appropriately effective interventions; everyone works together. The earlier we recognize an airway problem—and the earlier we implement intervention—the greater the mental and physical health benefits to the child for the rest of his or her life.

The Goal of The Airway Centric® Approach:

Focus on developing people's ability to breathe well while sleeping, in order to stop the epidemic of chronic diseases.

Our goal is to help you treat yourself and your family, and thus to start reversing the tide. Your health, your performance, and your life depend on your ability to breathe well.

Healthier lives through better breathing: that's Airway Centric®.

4

C H A P T E R

Kids: Breathing, Learning, & Sleeping

The following case study, "Finding Connor Deegan," is based on a story written by his mother, Valerie Deegan:

I can't tell our story without starting from the beginning. My son was never an "easy" child. From birth, he was always demanding, temperamental, and the complete opposite of eager-to-please. This behavior had slowly escalated, creating a blind tolerance. The year of 2011 was the straw that broke the camel's back.

My son was always one to be the center of attention, albeit negative attention. He was throwing temper tantrums in class and at home. He hated me and the world; the expression we heard the most was "I wish I was dead." He was always tearing up his homework and bullying someone. There seemed to be no rhyme or reason for his behavior. No trigger.

I could ask him to throw something out one day and he would do it without a fuss. But on other days, when given the same request, he would throw himself on the floor in a full tantrum at the age of 10. It would take him a couple of hours to compose himself once this happened.

His report card for 4th grade consisted of D's and F's, with a slew of negative comments from teachers. One teacher went so far as to say, "Your son may be 'gifted' but there is still something wrong with him. He doesn't belong in Challenge Core (the gifted program)."

Yes, my son was not behaving the same as the other kids. His inability to conform and to follow directions at home and at school was too much for everybody. The school was pushing me to put him on an IEP (Individual Education Program). Otherwise, they threatened to expel him from 4th grade.

Out of desperation, I signed the IEP and contacted several people to try to figure out, as one once put it, what was wrong with my son. First, I contacted his pediatrician. I requested allergy testing; a sleep study and anything else that may help us see if there was a medical issue. I also enrolled in a Parent-Child Interaction Therapy two times a week. The one decision I regret the most was the full psychological evaluation. It labeled him.

The psychological evaluation was performed on 12/14/11 before the allergy testing and sleep study results were available.

The sleep study results from Children's Hospital of Chicago were compiled and presented to me on 1/11/12. They were as follows:

- Snoring arousals
- Partial arousals
- Bruxism
- Increased upper airway resistance
- Obstructive sleep-disordered breathing

Allergy results from 2/16/12 stated that he has allergies to the following:

- Dogs (we have 2 large huskies)
- Cats (we have 2 domestics)
- Maple Trees (6 mature within 100 feet of our house)
- Walnut Trees (neighbor has 2 mature within 200 feet of our house)
- Cottonwood (passes 7 on his walk to school)
- Ash, Oak, Elm (again, all line the walk to school)

These allergies had no signs or symptoms; no itchy/watery eyes, sneezing, or post-nasal drip. There was nothing that would have alerted a parent that allergies were present.

It took the psychologist 4-6 weeks to put together the evaluation results. The psychological evaluation concluded (without taking into consideration the allergy test results and sleep study results) that my son is cognitively gifted and has ODD (oppositional defiant disorder). In order for the psychologist to include the "new" findings I would have to subject my son to another full evaluation.

By contrast, during our consultation with Dr Darius Loghmanee in the division of Pulmonary Medicine at Lurie Children's Hospital Chicago, he pointed us in the direction we needed to go to "fix" my son. He also prescribed some much needed allergy medication that would treat nasal congestion. He suggested that we contact Dr Kevin Boyd, DDS to see if my son qualifies for his case study.

So, how's a dentist going to fix behavior? Understanding the domino effect of undiagnosed allergies helps. The allergies caused his nasal passages to be chronically swollen. When someone cannot breathe through his nose, his only other option is the mouth. Mouth breathing 24 hours a day over a number of years takes a toll on the development of the mouth. A higher arch is developed in the palate; the jaw is no longer able to accommodate the tongue; the tonsils and adenoids work harder and can become enlarged. All of these things contribute to snoring. This is what I learned on our first visit to Dr Boyd: fix the mouth, snoring goes away, a full night's sleep is achieved, and behavioral dysfunction is remedied.

After 1 year of treatment with Dr Boyd, one tonsil and adenoidectomy, one frenulum-release by laser, a daily dose of allergy medication and I am able proudly to introduce you to my son.

Signs of Airway Obstruction:
» Mouth breathing
» Open or slack-mouthed posture
» Snoring or noisy sleep
» Night terrors
» Bed-wetting
» Chronic nasal discharge/ runny nose
» Chronic ear infections
» Dark circles or allergic "black eyes"
» Tossing, turning, thrashing and restless sleep
» Messy sheets and blankets
» Nail-biting
» Crooked teeth
» Frequent earaches
» Falling asleep in school
» Awakening feeling un-re-freshed

We found my son Connor. I knew he was there the whole time but we could not see him beyond his exhaustion.

My son's future looks bright. He has traded his D's and F's for 3 A's and 1 B. He's not perfect and can make some poor choices at times. He is still learning how to re-invent himself to get past being "that kid" at school. I am proud to report that he is succeeding.

Who knows if my son could be the catalyst that changes conventional thinking at his school? Because of this experience, maybe the teachers have learned to ask the parent of a struggling child, "Has your child been tested for allergies?" or "Have you considered having your child's sleep evaluated?"

Maybe, just maybe, because of the work Dr Boyd and Dr Loghmanee are doing, the medical world would prescribe both allergy test and sleep studies when a "behaviorally challenged" child enters grade school. In my humble opinion, the health of our country would greatly improve.

I will forever be grateful to Dr Loghmanee and Dr Boyd. They alone, with their forward thinking, bravery to act outside the parameters of what their colleagues expect from them, and questioning the big business of pharmaceuticals, have given my son back to me. They have brought peace to our house and joy to our hearts. They have given my son something I could not—the ability to sleep tight.

Thank You, Thank You, Thank You, Thank You, Thank You, Thank You, Thank You…a million times over![1]

(Note: Connor was treated by Airway Centric® dentist Dr Kevin Boyd.)

Sleep-Disordered Breathing in Kids

We all know how much kids need sleep, but it has to be the right kind of sleep. Just like adults, children need to breathe well while they sleep in order for their sleep to be restorative. Even more important for children, though, is deep, restorative sleep that promotes optimal brain development. Only through breathing well while sleeping can a child's brain develop to its maximum potential.

According to the American Academy of Sleep Medicine, sleep-disordered breathing causes disrupted and inefficient sleep, which in turn results in not only fatigue and daytime sleepiness, but also cognitive impairment and poor performance in school.[2] Even if a child gets to bed "early enough" then, they could still have problems with fatigue, focus, and learning.

---

1 The story of *Finding Connor Deegan* can be seen in video format here: http://aapmd.org/about-aapmd/aapmd-blog/entry/finding-connor-deegan.html

2 As referenced in Bonuck, Karen, and Roy Grant, "Sleep Problems and Early Developmental Delay: Implications for Early Intervention Programs," *Intellectual and Developmental Disabilities*, 2012, Vol. 50, No. 1, 41-52.

The problem is that many children develop mouth breathing, snoring, or even sleep apneas at a young age.[3] Surprisingly, airway-centered disorders resulting in sleep-disordered breathing (SDB) can start at birth, especially among premature babies.[4]

According to one researcher, about 10% of children snore, and roughly 2-4% have sleep apnea, which would mean, without counting mouth-breathers and hypopnea, at least 12-14% of children have some form of SDB.[5] Another study, which surveyed parents about a variety of SDBs including mouth breathing, showed that 4-11% of children have SDBs.[6] A study of 20,000 children in China found that 12% of children snored.[7]

The rates reported by the National Sleep Foundation are even higher. In a survey of parents, they found that 19% of preschoolers were reported as snoring a few times a week, and 19% of preschoolers also had difficulty waking up in the morning. In this same survey, 18% of school-aged children were reported to snore at least a few times a week, and 29% of school-aged children had difficulty waking up in the morning.[8]

3 Bonuck, Karen, et al, "Sleep-Disordered Breathing in a Population-Based Cohort: Behavioral Outcomes at 4 and 7 years," *Pediatrics*, March 5, 2012, http://pediatrics.aappublications.org/content/early/2012/02/29/peds.2011-1402.full.pdf+html

4 Huang, Yu-Shu, and Christian Guilleminault, "Pediatric Obstructive Sleep Apnea and the Critical Role of Oro-Facial Growth: Evidences," *Frontiers in Neurology*, 2012, 3:184, p. 9. http://www.ncbi.nlm.nih.gov/pmc/articles/PMC3551039/

5 http://www.livescience.com/18818-kids-sleep-breathing-behavioral-problems.html

6 Bonuck, Karen, and Roy Grant, "Sleep Problems and Early Developmental Delay: Implications for Early Intervention Programs," *Intellectual and Developmental Disabilities*, 2012, Vol. 50, No. 1, 41-52.

7 Li, Shenghui, Xinming Jin, Chonghuai Yan, Shenghu Wu, Fan Jiang, Xiaoming Shen, "Habitual Snoring in School-Aged Children: Environmental and Biological Predictors," *Respiratory Research* 2010, 11:144. http://respiratory-research.com/content/11/1/144/abstract

8 http://sleepfoundation.org/sites/default/files/FINAL%20SOF%202004.pdf

In the remarkable "Avon Longitudinal Study of Parents and Children," which started with over 8,000 infants just six months old and followed them for nearly seven years, researchers found that 10-21% of children aged 6-81 months snored.[9]

Clearly we have an epidemic of sleep-disordered breathing among children. Worse yet, the numbers are higher than was previously thought, and the trend has been consistently growing.

Snoring and mouth breathing are two primary indications of ACD as well as the two most prevalent forms of sleep-disordered breathing in children. When children are snoring or breathing through their mouths, their brains and bodies cannot develop correctly.

According to presenters at a recent conference on sleep and the importance of opening the airways, breathing through the mouth fails to accomplish five essential tasks that breathing through the nose achieves: humidifying the air; warming the air; filtering the air; accelerating the air; and releasing nitric oxide (NO), which kills dust mites and helps reduce inflammation.[10]

If you have children, we hope you are now wondering if your child could have ACD and sleep-disordered breathing. Listening to and observing how your child breathes while sleeping is the first step you as a parent can take in protecting your child's health. Signs of the possible presence of sleep-disordered breathing include: mouth breathing, snoring or noisy sleeping, bed-wetting, night terrors, open or slack-mouthed posture at rest, chronic nasal discharge or runny nose, chronic sinus infections, chronic ear infections, dark circles or allergic "black eyes," thrashing in the bed and restless sleep, messy bed sheets in the morning, nail-biting, and crooked teeth.

---

9 Bonuck, Karen, et al, "Sleep-Disordered Breathing in a Population-Based Cohort: Behavioral Outcomes at 4 and 7 years," *Pediatrics*, March 5, 2012, p. 2.

10 Dr Kevin Boyd, DDS, MS, and Dr Ben Miraglia, DDS, speaking at the AAPMD spring 2014 conference in Chicago, "The Silent Airway Connection: Its Impact on Development, Performance, and Health," http://aapmd.org/

Sleep, Brain Development, and Learning

Kids not only need a lot of sleep, they need a much higher percentage of deep sleep and REM sleep than adults. Newborns typically sleep 10.5 to 18 hours a day.[11] Newborns spend about 50% of their time sleeping in deep sleep (NREM, that is, non-rapid eye-movement) when the brain waves are slowest. Stage 3 NREM sleep is when the brain waves become delta waves, during which the body repairs and restores itself, bones and muscles are built, and the immune system is strengthened.

Non-REM Sleep	3 Stages	Transitioning from light sleep to slow-wave (deep sleep)
Stage N1	Transition to Sleep	Lasts about 5 minutes; eyes move slowly; muscle activity slows down; easily awakened
Stage N2	Light Sleep	First stage of true sleep; lasts 10-25 minutes; eye movement stops; heart rate slows; body temperature decreases
Stage N3	Deep Sleep	Difficult to awaken; if awakened, do not adjust immediately and often feel groggy and disoriented. Brain waves are extremely slow. Blood flow is directed away from brain and towards muscles, restoring physical energy.
REM Sleep		
REM	Dream Sleep	70-90 minutes after falling asleep; eyes move rapidly; heart rate and blood pressure increase, while breathing shallows; arms and legs are paralyzed; dreams are common

The other 50% of the time, newborns experience REM sleep (rapid eye movement), which is when dreaming occurs. During REM sleep, the brain waves indicate the brain is more alert (alpha), but major muscle groups in the body are effectively paralyzed. In comparison to newborns, adults spend only about 20% of the time

---

11 The National Sleep Foundation: http://sleepfoundation.org/sleep-topics/children-and-sleep

in REM sleep.[12] The quality of sleep matters as much as the amount of sleep. In order to attain and maintain deep NREM sleep, children must breathe well with open airways.

Researchers at the University of California, San Francisco studied sleep and brain development in young cats. They found that cats who were exposed to new environmental challenges and then allowed to sleep for six hours formed more brain connections than cats who were not allowed to sleep afterward.[13] Increasing the number of connections between neurons is referred to as brain plasticity, and plasticity increases primarily during deep sleep.[14]

Importantly, these deep-sleep stages are vital to the development of the prefrontal cortex, the area of the brain that consolidates new information and learning. Since children have to learn rapidly, especially during their early years and at school, sufficient deep sleep is essential to their brain's ability to learn and to remember.[15]

The prefrontal cortex, which does not fully develop until well into a person's 20s,[16] also provides the ability to plan, to reason, and to problem-solve, all essential skills for children to develop in order to function well in school and in life.[17] So, deep sleep, or NREM sleep, is essential to a child's ability to learn, to reason, and to problem-solve.

REM sleep is essential for young children as well. It helps form emotional memories, learn new skills like how to play a musical instrument, and enable decision-making.[18] Some researchers

---

12 http://www.webmd.com/sleep-disorders/excessive-sleepiness-10/sleep-101?page=2

13 http://issalab.uchicago.edu/papers/2.pdf

14 http://www.fi.edu/learn/brain/sleep.html

15 http://www.psychologytoday.com/blog/child-sleep-zzzs/201302/the-prefrontal-cortex-during-sleep

16 http://hrweb.mit.edu/worklife/youngadult/brain.html

17 http://brain.oxfordjournals.org/content/122/5/994.full Gerhand, Simon, "The Pre-Frontal Cortex – Executive and Cognitive Functions," The Oxford Journals, *Brain, a Journal of Neurology,* Vol. 122, Issue 5, pp. 994-995.

18 Stickgold, R., et al, "Sleep, Learning, and Dreams: Off-Line Memory Processing," Science 2 November 2001: 1052-1057 and http://www.fi.edu/learn/brain/sleep.html

believe that REM sleep is necessary in developing the capacity to deal with the stress of learning new skills and information.[19] Either way, children clearly need REM sleep.

One study of adults enrolled in an intensive language course found that they spent more time in REM sleep. The researchers theorized that REM sleep "played an essential role" in the acquisition of a new language.[20] If language acquisition is assisted by increased REM sleep, this would certainly explain why young children need so much more REM sleep than adults, since they are essentially learning a new language.

Researchers have also found that during the first five years of life, the human brain forms connections between the left and right hemispheres during sleep. Studying children ages 2, 3, and 5 years of age, researchers at the University of Colorado at Boulder found that these hemisphere connections increased as children got older, sometimes by up to 20%.[21]

This period of early childhood is critical in brain development, and sleep plays an important role in that development. A newborn's brain weighs only about 25% of an adult brain, but by age three a child's brain is 80-85% the size of an adult's, and by age five, a child's brain is 90% the size of an adult's.[22]

A newborn baby's brain already contains all the nerve cells, or neurons, it will ever need, but it continues to grow by adding millions of new synapses (the connections between brain cells), and by a process called myelination, which involves coating the nerve cells with fatty deposits. This fatty layer insulates brain cells,

19 http://healthysleep.med.harvard.edu/healthy/matters/benefits-of-sleep/learning-memory

20 http://healthysleep.med.harvard.edu/healthy/matters/benefits-of-sleep/learning-memory

21 http://www.sciencedaily.com/releases/2013/11/131120155215.htm , Salome Kurth, Peter Achermann, Thomas Rusterholz, Monique LeBourgeois. Development of Brain EEG Connectivity across Early Childhood: Does Sleep Play a Role? *Brain Sciences*, 2013; 3 (4): 1445 DOI: 10.3390/brainsci3041445

22 http://www.zerotothree.org/child-development/brain-development/faqs-on-the-brain.html

enabling them to communicate faster, which means speeding up the rate at which the brain processes information.[23]

Clearly then, the first five years are crucial to a child's brain development. The magnitude of brain development during early childhood suggests that this period represents the most important time to start preventing sleep-disordered breathing in order to protect the brain development of children during sleep. Addressing SDBs at this age will be most effective at preventing the epidemic of epigenetically derived chronic diseases for the rest of a child's life.

The Devastating Effects of SDBs in Children

The Division of Sleep Medicine at Harvard Medical School describes the impact of sleep deprivation. When people of all ages are sleep-deprived, they experience the following difficulties:

> **Having ACD** is like trying to breathe through a coffee stirrer instead of through a garden hose.

- Focus and attention diminish
- Vigilance—the ability to remain awake, alert, and attentive—is hampered
- Receiving information becomes more difficult
- Overload occurs – Over-worked neurons no longer function properly to coordinate information
- Decision-making ability declines because we have difficulty assessing and interpreting situations
- Planning becomes difficult
- Judgment is impaired
- Performance is affected because neurons do not fire optimally and muscles are not rested
- Internal synchronization is hampered – The body's organ systems are not synchronized
- Focus diminishes – Lapses of focus and daytime sleepiness can lead to accident or injury[24]

---

23 Ibid., and http://www.fcs.uga.edu/ext/bbb/brainTimeEarlyChild.php

24 http://healthysleep.med.harvard.edu/healthy/matters/benefits-of-sleep/learning-memory

With regard to children, because their brains are still developing, the problems caused by sleep deprivation and sleep-disordered breathing are even greater. To understand how a blocked airway affects children so dramatically, try placing your hand over your nose and mouth, pressing somewhat hard, while trying to breathe for one minute. Even if you can get a little air around and through the cracks between your fingers, notice how hard it becomes to get a good, deep breath. This is what sleeping with a partially blocked airway (ACD) feels like. Having ACD is like trying to breathe through a tiny coffee stirrer instead of through a garden hose.

Under such conditions during sleep, the brain unconsciously recognizes that it is not getting enough oxygen, and it signals that a crisis is occurring. The EEG pattern is immediately changed, often arousing a sleeper from deep, delta sleep right up to alpha (light) sleep. The chemical signals in the brain that go along with that sense of crisis cause a cascade of reactions in the brain's chemistry. These chemical changes signal a stress response throughout the body.[25]

In other words, having difficulty breathing during sleep makes the brain think it is threatened. It is as if that next breath may never come! That threatened brain immediately turns on all of the body's survival instincts, the fight-or-flight response. It tells the adrenal glands to release a flood of the stress hormone, adrenaline, putting us into full panic mode.

Over time, that adrenaline has toxic effects and causes the body's immune responses to run wild and create inflammation throughout the body. When interrupted by apnea, snoring and other breathing disorders, the sleep process becomes a time of crisis rather a time of rest, repair and restoration. Your brain, its messenger chemicals (neurotransmitters) and immune system are in a state of red alert and they often stay that way.

For children, this state of alert for the brain and body, along with hypoxia (lack of oxygen), excess carbon dioxide, and sleep fragmentation, can lead to symptoms of attention deficit hyperac-

---

25 Schraufnagel, Dean E., *Breathing In America: Diseases, Progress, and Hope,* The American Thoracic Society, 2010, p. 241. http://www.thoracic.org/education/breathing-in-america/resources/chapter-23-sleep-disordered-breathing.pdf

tivity disorder (ADHD), hyperactivity, learning disabilities, anxiety, depression, lack of social coping skills, and peer-related problems including aggressive behavior.

According to researcher Dr Karen Bonuck of the Albert Einstein College of Medicine, sleep-disordered breathing can damage the prefrontal cortex of children, resulting in speech and language issues, including the impairment of verbal fluency and the "ability to use verbal cues to direct or organize behavior."[26] Some of these deficits may be reversed as sleep-disordered breathing is treated,[27] although, as Bonuck notes in the journal *Pediatrics*, some of the neurological effects of SDBs may be irreversible.[28]

One of these neurological deficits is a potentially lower IQ. Researchers in Tucson studied the relationship between sleep apnea in children and their ability to learn, to remember, and to perform. Children with higher rates of sleep-disordered breathing performed lower on tests of ability to learn, to remember, and to perform, and tended to have lower IQs overall.[29]

> **Obstructive Sleep Apnea** may reduce a child's IQ by as much as 10 points.

These brain deficits caused by sleep-disordered breathing begin in very young children, from infancy through the pre-school years. This means that intervening very early in a child's life to prevent SDBs is essential to their future health and their ability to learn as

---

26 Bonuck, Karen, and Roy Grant, "Sleep Problems and Early Developmental Delay: Implications for Early Intervention Programs," *Intellectual and Developmental Disabilities*, 2012, Vol. 50, No. 1, p. 43.

27 Ibid.

28 Bonuck, Karen, et al, "Sleep-Disordered Breathing in a Population-Based Cohort: Behavioral Outcomes at 4 and 7 years," *Pediatrics*, March 5, 2012, p. 2.

29 Kaemingk, KL et al, "Learning in Children and Sleep-Disordered Breathing: Findings of the Tucson's Children's Assessment of Sleep Apnea (TuCASA) Prospective Cohort Study," *Journal of the International Neuropsychological Society*, 2003, Nov; 9 (7): 1016-26. http://www.ncbi.nlm.nih.gov/pubmed/14738283

early as the first year of life. In her study,[30] Bonuck recommends intervention for SDBs during the first year.

As Dr Stephen Sheldon, Professor of Pediatrics at Northwestern University and Director of the Sleep Medicine Center at Lurie Children's Hospital in Chicago states, in reference to the relationship between children's sleep and their brain health: "We have to diagnose early because of oxygen deprivation... If we don't fix it by then [age 5], it's going to be broken, and it's going to be broken for good."

Studies looking at school-aged children show that children with even mild to moderate sleep-disordered breathing—from snoring to obstructive sleep apnea—have more behavioral problems in school than children who don't have SDBs. One study of middle school children found that "children with lower academic performance in middle school are more likely to have snored during early childhood... compared with better performing schoolmates."[31]

Again, this study implies that the effects of SDBs while children are young are not entirely reversible, especially if they are not treated at a young age. In fact, researcher David Gozal suggests that young children with SDBs may develop a "learning debt" that may "hamper subsequent school performance."[32] Gozal found that obstructive sleep apnea may reduce a child's IQ on average by 10 points.

One of the landmark studies of children and sleep-disordered-breathing is the Avon Longitudinal Study by Dr Karen Bonuck. Bonuck's study followed over 11,000 children for a period of seven years from birth onward. What Bonuck and her colleagues found provides a very clear association between sleep-disordered breathing (SDBs) and high rates of ADHD, along with other problems such as anxiety, depression, and aggressive behavior.

---

30 Ibid, p. 8.

31 Gozal, David, and Dennis W. Pope, Jr., "Snoring During Early Childhood and Academic Performance at ages Thirteen to Fourteen Years," *Pediatrics* 2001, 107:6, 1394-1399.

32 Ibid.

First of all, Bonuck's study found that SDBs are "relatively common in childhood."[33] The study relied on parents to report snoring, mouth breathing, and apneas in children, noting that snoring was probably the easiest form of SDB for parents to observe. Based on parents' reports, the study found that "the prevalence of habitual snoring ranged from 10-21% from 6-81 months."[34] Moreover, the percentage of children who never showed signs of SDBs was only 45%.[35]

Second, and most important, the Bonuck study found that "sleep-disordered breathing was associated with 40% and 60% more behavioral difficulties at 4 and 7 years respectively." By age four, children with symptoms of SDBs were 20-60% more likely to exhibit behavior problems. By age seven, children with SDBs were 40-100% more likely to exhibit behavior problems that fit clinical diagnoses.[36]

In the realm of behavior problems, SDBs are most strongly linked to inattentiveness and hyperactivity. However, children with sleep-disordered breathing also were far more likely to experience anxiety and depression, have problems getting along with their peers, display aggressive behavior and breaking of rules, and these same children were far less likely to engage in positive social behaviors such as sharing and helping.

> **By age four**, children with symptoms of SDBs were 20-60% more likely to exhibit behavior problems. By age seven, children with SDBs were 40-100% more likely to exhibit behavior problems that fit clinical diagnoses.

The SDBs associated with behavior problems at age 4 were just as valid at predicting problems at age 7. The children who had the highest levels of mouth breathing, snoring, and apneas

---

33 Bonuck, Karen, Katherine Freeman, Ronald D. Chervin, and Linzhi Xu, "Sleep-Disordered Breathing in a Population-Based Cohort: Behavioral Outcomes at 4 and 7 Years," Pediatrics, March 5, 2012, p. 8. http://pediatrics.aappublications.org/content/early/2012/02/29/peds.2011-1402.full.pdf+html

34 Ibid.

35 Ibid., p. 3.

36 Ibid., p. 5.

throughout the study, and whose symptoms peaked at 30 months, experienced the most significant long-term effects. However, even the children whose SDB symptoms peaked as young as 6 months and 18 months but then reduced in severity, experienced 40% and 50% increased likelihood of behavioral problems, respectively.[37]

Even a child who temporarily experiences SDBs at age 6 months is 40% more likely to have behavior issues such as ADHD, anxiety or aggression at age four or seven. Given this statistic, early intervention to treat SDBs becomes imperative.

What this means is that if a child shows signs of SDBs at age 6 months, even if the SDBs are corrected, because the brain is developing so rapidly at this young age, the SDBs often permanently affected the child.[38] A baby who experiences temporary breathing issues during sleep, whether stuffy nose and mouth breathing or snoring at age six months, is 40% more likely to have behavioral problems such as ADHD at age 4 or 7. Given this sobering statistic, early intervention to treat SDBs becomes imperative, whether the goal is treatment or prevention.[39]

A child already diagnosed with ADHD at age 2 or 3 would be well served to have an evaluation of the following: his/her sleep, ability to breathe through the nose, facial tone, jaw development, and overall airway openness. This is particularly important in light of the fact that the Centers for Disease Control found that 100,000 toddlers in the U.S. are being treated with ADHD medications like Ritalin and Adderall. These medications have not even been tested on children under 4, nor are they recommended for children under the age of 4. Unfortunately, children on Medicaid are even more likely to be placed on these medications, but preventing sleep-disordered breathing could be just what these children need most in order to succeed in school and in life.[40]

What about down the road, as the child matures? Some researchers are starting to question whether or not these early issues

---

37 Ibid., p. 7.

38 Ibid., p. 7.

39 Ibid., p. 9.

40 http://www.nytimes.com/2014/05/17/us/among-experts-scrutiny-of-attention-disorder-diagnoses-in-2-and-3-year-olds.html?_r=0

with sleep-disordered breathing—that lead to anxiety, aggression, peer-to-peer difficulties, and depression—may be at the root of the psycho-emotional problems experienced by teenagers. Although adolescents experience that legendary roller-coaster ride of emotions due to other factors such as hormonal fluctuations, and not all teens are mouth-breathers, it would seem likely that undiagnosed, untreated breathing disorders continue to have an impact in teen years, and this warrants further study—especially in this troubling age of tragic school shootings. Because these neurological deficits from SDBs may be permanent, and because SDBs cause brain chemical imbalances, SDBs in children may lead to long term problems such as anxiety, lack of social connection, and depression. We can't afford to ignore all the possibilities.

This question of causality in teen violence was raised by two presenters at the April, 2014, meeting of the American Academy of Physiological Medicine and Dentistry in Chicago, of which we were co-hosts. Researcher Dr William Walsh of the Walsh Research Institute near Chicago raised the question about sleep-disordered breathing and the attendant neurochemical imbalances vis a vis school-shooters. And Dr Ben Miraglia, DDS, of Mt. Kisco, New York, showed a slide of Adam Lanza, the school-shooter in Newtown, Connecticut, surmising, based on this, that he had blockage of his airway. Although it is impossible to know now, it is important to ask the questions.

The Physical Effects

In addition to these psychological issues, a child with sleep-disordered breathing is likely to develop obesity and a variety of physical health issues as well. For instance, Dr David Gozal, a leading researcher on pediatric sleep medicine in Chicago, IL, studied the possible link between sleep-disordered breathing and the development of cardiovascular disease in children. Gozal found that children with obstructive sleep apnea (OSA) in fact developed some physiological changes that often lead to heart disease. Different studies found that OSA in children could lead to decreased heart rate variability, increased systemic inflammation, and endothelial dysfunction, all of which contribute to increased cardiovascular risks. The good news is that children who had their tonsils and adenoids removed (adenotonsillectomy, or AT) experienced some reversal of these negative trends.[41]

Gozal also conducted research showing that children with OSA have a higher rate of immune system disruption, causing increased systemic inflammation. DNA methylation in children with OSA leads to epigenetic changes, which keep the immune system in "constant overdrive, putting stress on the body's organs."[42] Many children with OSA also had higher levels of high-sensitivity C-reactive Protein (hsCRP), and those with both high levels of hsCRP and OSA had higher rates of DNA methylation. The more severe cases of sleep apnea had the highest rates of DNA methylation, thus showing that OSA in children can indicate increased risk of inflammation, compromised immune system, and greater stress on the body's major organs.[43]

Finally, let's consider children who died suddenly of unexplained causes, often in their sleep. To investigate sleep-disordered breathing and its impact on children, researchers Rambaud and Guilleminault studied two groups: 1) seven infants and children who died sudden deaths, and 2) seven live children who had sleep-disordered breathing.

All the children were found to have abnormal enlargement of the soft tissues in their upper airways as well as abnormal facial development in the form of small, narrow, and highly arched palates, and several of the children had acute, often mild rhinitis.[44] The significance of Rambaud and Guilleminault's study is that every child who died abruptly had the kind of abnormal facial development that leads to blocked airways, swelling of the nasal passages, and sleep-disordered breathing.

---

41 Bhattacharjee, Rakesh, MD and David Gozal MD, FCCP, "Pediatric Sleep Apnea: The Brain-Heart Connection," *Chest*. May 2011; 139 (5):977-979. http://www.ncbi.nlm.nih.gov/pmc/articles/PMC3087460/

42 Wood, Matt, "The Deep Impact of Childhood Sleep Apnea," *Science Life*, The University of Chicago Medicine and Biological Sciences, March 1, 2012.

43 Ibid.

44 Rambaud, Caroline, and Christian Guilleminault, "Death, naso-maxillary complex, and sleep in young children," *European Journal of Pediatrics*, September 2012, Volume 171, Issue 9, pp. 1349-1358.

In a recent lecture, researcher Kevin Boyd, DDS, MS, referenced unexplained cases of SIDS (Sudden Infant Death Syndrome), proposing that these might be attributed to the infants' high, narrow palates—the kind of mouth and jaw structure that leads to sleep-disordered breathing.[45]

A final concern about children and sleep-disordered breathing is that the risk of SDBs is higher for children who are obese, children of parents who smoke, and African-American children.[46] Further research is needed to assess the causes and preventions of any and all elevated risk factors for SDBs in children because their very lives depend on it.

---

45 Kevin Boyd, DDS, MS, in a lecture on "Malocclusion – Risk Factor for Obstructive Sleep Apnea (OSA) in Children: A Darwinian Perspective," at the April 2014 meeting of the AAPMD in Chicago.

46 Redline, Susan, et al, "Risk Factors for Sleep-Disordered Breathing in Children, Associations with Obesity, Race, and Respiratory Problems," *American Journal of Respiratory and Critical Care Medicine*, Vol. 159, No. 5 (1999), pp. 1527-1532. http://www.atsjournals.org/doi/abs/10.1164/ajrccm.159.5.9809079#.UwvJEvRDuT8 and for an association between snoring in children and the presence of an adult smoking in the home, please see: http://www.fi.edu/learn/brain/sleep.html

Part II - Compromised Airways: A Lifelong Problem

5

C H A P T E R

Your Child's Face: Preventing Life-Long Problems

Facial Development in Children

As children grow in the womb and after birth, their jaws develop along with their entire skull and the muscles of their face, head, and neck. Everything links together as it grows. So what affects the muscles affects the jaws, neck, and head as well.

During development, form follows function. In the case of developing faces, noses, and jaws, the way the muscles of the mouth and face are used help create the shape of the jaws and face, because the stress of using the muscles causes bone to be deposited along the sutures of the bones, which lengthens and widens the jaws and cheekbones.

Ideally, jaws should be wide and U-shaped. In recent decades, though, because of the various epigenetic effects discussed previously, our jaws have become smaller, crowding the space for our teeth so they become crooked, jaws often develop overbites or are pushed backwards (retruded), and even open-mouthed slack jaws result. Today, it is common to see V-shaped jaws that create a high narrow palate and obstructed nasal passages.

Joanne, age 14, is a typical kid, doing well in school, but she had TMJ pain (pain in her jaw joints). Her jaws would click and also lock up after eating or awakening. She clenched her teeth at night and had daily headaches. She also had back pain. Her parents brought her to Dr Michael Gelb, DDS.

Joanne has large tonsils, as well as the typical forward head posture of a mouth breather, rounded shoulders, slouched posture, and a sway back. Dr Gelb sent her to a pediatric rheumatologist to rule out any autoimmune disorders as potential causes of her joint pain. He fitted Joanne with a night-bite appliance with a ramp to bring her jaw forward at night. This has eliminated the clicking. Bringing her jaws forward and expansion of her palate will come next in her treatment plan.

The reason that optimal facial formation consists of wide, U-shaped jaws (aka the maxilla and mandible) is that it leads to a better bite (no malocclusion) as well as a wide enough nose to create open nasal passages that promote nasal breathing, and a tongue that has plenty of room to rest in the mouth. In other words, if the mouth is the parking garage, there will be plenty of room to park the tongue without it getting scallops on the side edges from pressing against the teeth.

In addition, there is so-called "proper oral rest posture": breathing through the nose, the teeth slightly apart, and the tongue resting or pressing lightly on the roof of the mouth (the palate).

A number of factors affect proper oral rest posture, which includes the whole position of the neck and head.[1] Many children have a forward-head posture, where the ears no longer align directly above the shoulders, and this misalignment signals improper oral rest posture. The forward-head posture is common among mouth-breathers, and typically includes a slouched standing position and sway back as well.

As we look at the faces of children today, we see many children mouth breathing with slack-jaws, puffed out lips that lack muscle tone, and cheeks that melt directly into the neck with no prominent

---

1 According to personal communication from Paula Fabbie, OMT, a highly skilled Orofacial Myofunctional Therapist, oral rest posture involves many factors, and is not as simple as placing the tongue up against the palate, breathing through the nose, and keeping the lips together.

cheekbone definition. Such facial slackness is partly due to lack of muscle tone, or hypotonia. Many premature babies are born with hypotonia, but hypotonia can be present at all ages, and is often linked to sleep-disordered breathing.[2]

Factors that contribute to poor facial development:
» Bottle-feeding
» Weaning to soft foods
» Thumb-sucking
» Pacifier Use
» Mouth breathing

Remember, these facial characteristics are not genetic; they are epigenetic changes, influenced by a variety of environmental factors. For instance, babies who are born premature tend to have narrow arches and high-vaulted palates. Bottle-feeding furthers such malformations because of inadequate use of muscles for sucking and swallowing. Soft foods such as baby cereals hinder proper facial development by minimizing the muscle use and development that chewing promotes. Thumb-sucking and pacifier use can contribute to poor facial development as well. Mouth breathing strongly contributes to the formation of these abnormal facial features.

Breastfeeding, especially for the "normative" or ancestral pattern of 3+ years, along with weaning babies to chewable foods, develops the jaw most fully.

Proper facial development is essential for proper breathing, deep sleep, and good health.

But this poor epigenetic development begins in utero. Ultrasound images of babies in the womb can show whether or not a child's jaw is already retrognathic (positioned backwards), as well as whether or not the child is sucking her thumb. For more on the importance of a baby's development in utero, please read the section on pregnancy in Chapter 7.

The good news is that proper orofacial development can begin at birth, and unhealthy orofacial development can be treated beginning at birth. Perhaps someday treatment will be available in utero as well.

---

2 Huang, Yu-Shu, and Christian Guilleminault, "Pediatric Obstructive Sleep Apnea and the Critical Role of Oral-Facial Growth: Evidences," *Frontiers in Neurology,* 2012; 3: 184. http://www.ncbi.nlm.nih.gov/pmc/articles/PMC3551039/#B33

Tonsils and Adenoids

Health care providers are in the process of going full circle on the subject of the removal of tonsils and adenoids in children. Tonsils are lymphatic tissue on each side at the back of the throat, and adenoids are small lymphatic tissue masses a little higher up where the nasal passages meet the throat.

Fifty or more years ago, it was common practice to remove tonsils and adenoids at the first sign of infection. Then medical science discovered that these tiny pieces of tissue at the back of the throat are an important component of the immune system. Tonsils and adenoids are composed of lymphatic tissue that filters out viruses and bacteria and that produces antibodies to fight off infection. So, for the last two or three decades, pediatricians have recommended that tonsils and adenoids be left in, even when a child has recurrent throat infections.

Now, however, we are able to detect the degree to which tonsils and adenoids block off a child's airway, using cephalometric X-rays and 3D-CT images of the upper airway. Tonsils and adenoids can be graded on a scale of 1 to 4 to determine how much blockage they cause. Because enlarged tonsils and adenoids can contribute to blocked airways and therefore create or worsen sleep-disordered breathing, having a child's tonsils and adenoids evaluated by an ENT (Ear, Nose, and Throat doctor) is very important.

In fact, when children breathe through their mouths during sleep, the increased turbulence of the breath going directly into the throat instead of going first through the nose causes inflammation and potentially enlargement of the tonsils and adenoids.[3]

A vicious cycle is created: mouth breathing doesn't filter out germs and fails to humidify the air. The dry air leads to enlarged adenoids and tonsils, and the germs can infect them. The child who breathes through his or her mouth and has enlarged tonsils and adenoids experiences more sleep-disordered breathing, which can lead to compromised immunity, increasing the likelihood of colds and sore throats, which in turn increases the likelihood of mouth breathing and swollen tonsils, and on and on.

---

3 Huang and Guilleminault, 2012.

Complicating matters further, both tonsils and adenoids grow proportionately faster than the child's body in the pre-school years. In fact, the size of tonsils and adenoids peaks between the ages of 4 and 8,[4] well before the airway finishes developing, making their size, relative to a young child's throat, appear much greater than their actual size. However, tonsils and adenoids begin to shrink during the teen years, causing less blockage of the airway from puberty onward.

For this reason, many pediatricians advise the parents to "wait and see," instead of having their child's tonsils removed. Of course, many parents would prefer to watch and wait before opting for surgery. While waiting may seem like a better option than putting a child through supposedly "unnecessary" surgery, this may be terribly flawed thinking that can have long-term repercussions throughout the child's life.

> **Emily**, who came in at age 11, used to sleep walk and sleep-talk. Her parents brought her to Dr Michael Gelb because she had clicking in her jaw for a year, along with jaw tenderness and headaches.
>
> After several months of treatment, bringing her jaw out and to the left (it was off-center before), Emily no longer sleep-walks or talks, has no more clicking, and her headaches are better. She used to be "hyper and have trouble concentrating," but now she is less "hyper." Her mother now says she is "doing well."

In fact, researchers have found that adenotonsillectomy (or AT, removal of the tonsils and adenoids) can help young children reduce symptoms of obstructive sleep apnea. Among non-obese children, 51% of children had a complete resolution of SDBs after having an AT. Among obese children, the rates of success were lower.[5] However, because young children are so vulnerable to permanent brain deficits due to SDBs, and because young children's tonsils and adenoids tend to be proportionally so much larger, having an adenotonsillectomy represents a potentially vital step to protecting their brains at a young age.

---

4 Ackay, Ahmet, et al., "Variation in Tonsil Size in 4- to 17-Year-Old Schoolchildren," *Journal of Otolaryngology*, August 2006, Vol. 35, Issue 4, pp.270-274.

5 Huang and Guilleminault, 2012.

One study found that children showed no SDBs and no neurocognitive deficits both 3 months and 6 months after having their

---

Zoe, age 12, used to have stamina problems and had low muscle tone, so it was hard to keep her teeth together. She started treatments with Dr Jill Meyer-Hindin around age 8. She worked with an OMT (oro-facial myofunctional therapist) and was fitted with a Biobloc appliance. Now, her cephalometric X-ray (Ceph) shows that she does have a bigger airway, and she reportedly gets enough air.

Her parents report that she is doing better with her swimming—she's powerful and goes pretty fast, and Dr Jill Meyer-Hindin believes it's because Zoe breathes better. Dr Meyer-Hindin reports that Zoe was fidgety when she first came in; however, she is visibly less fidgety now.

Zoe's younger brother Noah, age 8, was breastfed for 18 months. Noah had a frenectomy. Dr Meyer-Hindin has also fitted him with a palate expander, retainer, then Biobloc. Noah reports that his least favorite is Biobloc, because "it hurts at first when you put it in, and you have to keep your teeth together." Noah also doesn't like "wasting time" three times a day to rinse his retainer.

We believe that parents need to know that treatment isn't necessarily easy, and that kids have to be compliant for treatment to work. Noah and Zoe's parents are committed to providing the best treatment for their children.

Parents will do well to remember that a couple of years of treatment could make a dramatic difference, positively shaping the rest of a child's life.

---

tonsils removed, thus showing the temporary resolution of sleep-disordered breathing that is so important for protecting their brains. However, after 5 years, 40% of the children again had sleep-disordered breathing and had developed abnormal neurocognitive scores.[6]

Fortunately, the researchers found that other modes of treatment following AT can help create long-term resolution of SDBs. Specifically, Huang and Guilleminault found that the combination of orthodontic work such as rapid maxillary expansion (RME) and orofacial

---

6 Ibid.

myofunctional therapy (OMT) can resolve both facial abnormalities and sleep-disordered breathing in children.[7]

The researchers found, however, that if children did not complete their myofunctional therapy, their hypotonia did not improve, resulting in their continuation of or relapse into mouth breathing.[8] This research thus emphasizes the importance of an interdisciplinary approach to treating SDBs in children, including removing tonsils and adenoids, orthodontic work that consists of "guided appliance therapy"[9] to open the airway, and orofacial myofunctional therapy.[10]

In his book, *Why? African American Children Cannot Read,* Dr Philip W. Cooper, Jr. shares a study that shows the elevated prevalence of sleep-disordered breathing among African-American children, noting that this is approximately the same percentage of children who struggle and have difficulties in school. Cooper also shares case studies of African-American children who had adenotonsillectomies and the impact on their education. For a child who was diagnosed early with OSA, the results were remarkable, leading the child to achieve at grade level. For a child who was diagnosed at a later age, the surgery resulted in improvements, but left long-term learning deficits because the neurocognitive damage from lack of oxygen during sleep had already occurred.[11]

For the sake of all children who deserve the ability to succeed in school and in life, pediatricians and dental health professionals need to be screening for any and all forms of airway-centered disorders and sleep-disordered breathing.

---

7 Ibid.

8 Ibid.

9 Dr Ben Miraglia, DDS, Miraglia Interceptive Orthodontics of New York.

10 For more information on the importance of OMT and the availability of practitioners, please see both of these sites: The Academy of Applied Myofunctional Sciences, http://aamsinfo.net/ and The International Association of Orofacial Myologists, http://www.iaom.com/IAOM/

11 Cooper, Philip W., Jr., DDS, Why African American Children Can Not Read, *iUniverse*, 2009, pp. 24 and 30.

Preventing, Diagnosing, and Treating SDBs in Children

Pediatric Case Study:

Meet Stefano, ten years old and in the late stages of having his airway opened and his jaws brought forward through orthotropics.

When Stefano was a baby, he nursed every two hours, because his parents did not realize he was tongue-tied. His parents researched everything. "We've seen other dentists and their methods, but we weren't convinced."

Then they met Dr Jill Meyer-Hindin, who uses Biobloc appliances to accomplish orthotropic expansion of the maxilla and mandible, bringing both jaws forward. Dr Meyer-Hindin was trained by Dr William M. Hang, one of the world's two foremost experts in orthotropics. Dr Jill explains her process with Stefano: "they <the other dentists> did not expand him as much as he needed. We expanded first, then brought the teeth forward, and then the biobloc goes up here <top of palate> and he bites here <with appliance in>. He has to speak with his teeth together for the condyle to come forward for the bone to remodel. He <also> had a frenectomy."

The results?

Dr Jill: "He's sleeping better, he used to be fidgety. He used to have just one REM sleep per night. He was also tired, and had black circles under the eyes. He's doing better now."

Stefano's Dad: "He tossed and turned and had restless leg syndrome—which is now gone."

Stefano confirmed that it's now easier to do better in school, and that wearing the special retainer helps him feel calmer, play soccer better, and he finds it easier to be still.

Choices we make for our kids and ourselves can improve chances of experiencing unobstructed breathing, a good night's sleep, healthy development, and a better life.

So that you have the information you need to take charge of your child's overall well-being, we present below several choices you can make to enable your child to be healthy, intelligent, self-controlled, happy, and able to succeed in school and in life. You have the power to take action to improve your child's life at every step.

» **Action: Healthy pregnancy.** We will discuss this more in the chapter on women and SDBs, because a healthy mom is better able to give birth to a healthy baby.

» **Action: Breastfeeding.** In 1987, researchers found that the longer the duration of breastfeeding, the lower the incidence of malocclusion. They also found that bottle-feeding created what's called "forward tongue thrust," which in turn contributes to bad bites (malocclusion) and difficulties swallowing. With longer durations of breastfeeding, they found reductions in tongue thrusting.[12]

One of the primary means of preventing SDBs in children is breastfeeding. When a child breastfeeds, the mother's nipple is pulled into the mouth and pressed up against the palate. Both the work of the child's muscles in the mouth and tongue and the pressure on the palate function to prompt more bone to be deposited along the suture lines of the mouth, thus widening both the maxilla and the mandible.

To breastfeed, a child needs the ability to suck, swallow, and breathe through the nose all at the same time. This can be hard or even impossible for premature infants and other babies with hypotonia. Orofacial myofunctional therapy can help increase muscle tone, but the window of opportunity to start breastfeeding is so short that many babies who can't seem to breastfeed are bottle fed instead.

For working moms today, it can be very difficult to breastfeed more than a few weeks. While we understand how challenging this may be, we recommend a minimum of six months and preferably much longer, if possible, for proper facial development. Breastfeeding helps a baby's jaw and breathing mechanisms develop in ways that prevent sleep-disordered breathing throughout life.

One of the difficulties that mothers and babies sometimes experience while breastfeeding is the double-whammy of the baby having difficulty latching onto the nipple, combined with

12 Labbok, M., et al, "Does Breastfeeding Protect Against Malocclusion?" *American Journal of Preventive Medicine*, 1987, 3 (4): 227-32.

extreme pain for the mother in her nipple and breast. When a baby is tongue-tied, the baby is unable to stick out its tongue while latching onto the breast, so it latches with its hard gums instead. This can cause the mother to feel severe pain, often making it too painful to breastfeed.

If a baby has a hard time breastfeeding, it is essential to see if the baby has ankyloglossia, or a tongue-tie. Many lactation consultants are trained to identify ankyloglossia. Orofacial myologists, or orofacial myofunctional therapists are also able to recognize the various forms of tongue-ties.

If breastfeeding is not possible, special "slow-flow, orthodontic" nipples are available to simulate the kind of work a baby has to do when nursing on the breast. If your baby is struggling to suck and getting frustrated, please consider having your baby evaluated for low muscle tone by an orofacial myofunctional therapist (OMT).

» **Action: Orofacial myofunctional therapy.** If your baby is having trouble breastfeeding or bottle-feeding, consulting with a lactation specialist while your child is an infant can help resolve the issues. If you feel stressed about your baby's struggle to nurse, it is vitally important that you have your child evaluated for poor facial muscle tone, or hypotonia.

For toddlers, preschoolers, and older children, orofacial my-ofunctional therapy can provide your child with simple, fun exercises to increase their ability to suck, swallow, breathe, chew, and speak well. An OMT will also teach your child proper oral rest posture, which helps develop nasal breathing and better facial development.

In one pediatric dental office, children as young as eighteen months are taught proper oral rest posture, and the whole family is educated about issues and exercises for the face and mouth to develop properly so that children will be able to breathe and sleep and live well.[13]

---

13 Dr Hila Robbins, DDS, www.lakidsdentist.com, personal communication.

» **Action: Frenulum release, (or frenotomy, or frenectomy).** If muscle tone is not your baby's issue when trying to nurse, a tight or restricted frenulum might be. "Tongue-tied" is the term we commonly use for people whose tongues have a tight frenulum that restricts their ability to move the tongue in any direction. A baby with a tight frenulum is unable to latch on and breastfeed properly. A tight frenulum leads to problems sucking, chewing, swallowing, and sometimes with speech as well. A tight frenulum can lead to poor orofacial development, including lack of development of the upper palate due to the tongue resting low in the mouth—which means it's also pressing backwards in the throat, and partially blocking the airway. If left untreated, a tight frenulum can lead not only to SDBs including sleep apnea, but also to musculoskeletal pain and problems in the jaw, head, neck and beyond.[14]

Because releasing the frenulum is so essential to a child's health, legislators in Brazil passed a law in 2014 stating that all newborn babies' tongues must be examined to see if they need a frenectomy, or tongue-tie release.

» **Action: Avoid pacifier use and prevent thumb-sucking.** Both of these practices encourage the palate to develop in that high V-shape, which makes breathing through the nasal passages difficult and aggravates airway obstruction. Thumb-sucking and the need for pacifiers are responses to stress and the child's instinctive desire to seek comfort. There is a wide variety of stress reduction methods for children and methods to stop thumb-sucking and dependence on pacifiers. In the case of pacifiers, we recommend that you avoid using them, period.

» **Action: Baby-led weaning.** Earlier, we mentioned that the Industrial Revolution introduced soft foods, including soft baby cereals, and that this largely contributed to the narrowing of our jaws and airways, so you know that introducing only soft foods to a baby or young child will not help their jaws and faces

---

14 Paula Fabbie, OMT, personal conversation on August 2, 2014, based on her own case studies, training, and years of experience.

develop properly. Yet, that is exactly what our culture has taught us to do.

There is now a movement called "baby-led weaning" (and also a book by that title), which helps us return to ancient feeding patterns. First, one breastfeeds as long as possible, and delays introducing other foods as long as possible, at least until the baby is 6 months old. Baby-led weaning means following what a child is ready to eat, so ideally one allows the child to eat when they start reaching for food and putting it in their mouths. Secondly, one gives the child choices, including foods that help them develop their chewing abilities, such as steamed carrots, sticks of raw cucumber or sticks of cheese. This approach empowers the baby in many ways, and because the child is self-feeding, orofacial development is enhanced along with fine motor coordination and hand-eye coordination.[15]

» **Action: Treat allergies and asthma.** If your child has any obvious breathing and airway issues such as nasal congestion, runny nose, sneezing, or asthma, we recommend that you get your child tested for allergies and evaluated by the pediatrician and an Ear, Nose, and Throat doctor as well. Any stuffiness of their nose at night can contribute to reducing the amount of oxygen they receive while sleeping.

» **Action: Avoid junk food.** Junk food creates a vicious circle. A child who is not sleeping well will crave sugar and carbohydrates or other unhealthy foods. For a short time, she feels better as the food revs up her body. But when blood sugar inevitably crashes, she gets tired, sleepy and cranky and craves more carbohydrates to restore the sugar high.

Diets high in simple carbohydrates like juice drinks, crackers, cookies, sugary cereals and even soft drinks lead to multiple metabolic problems, not the least of which are obesity and Type 2 diabetes. (So, yes, we are dentists, and we also don't

---

15 For more information, see, for instance, *Baby-Led Weaning, The Essential Guide to Introducing Solid Foods and Helping Your Baby Grow Up a Happy and confident Eater*, Gill Rapley and Tracey Murkett, (New York: The Experiment, LLC) 2010.

want your kids eating and drinking sugary foods and soft drinks because it will cause cavities!)

It's essential to interrupt the vicious cycle, because not only does poor sleep lead to carb cravings, but also the resulting obesity in turn increases sleep problems, especially SDBs. Remember, the prevalence of sleep apnea in overweight and obese children is much higher, so not only are they prone to health issues, but most likely learning issues as well.

» **Action: Epiglottis check.** For some children, this may be an important airway issue. Between the ages of six months and one year, a child's epiglottis descends. This flap of tissues contracts upon swallowing, preventing food or liquids from entering the windpipe. This can create another potential blockage to the airway. In some cases, surgery to remove a portion of the epiglottis may help clear a child's airway.

» **Action: Be aware of and reduce exposure to environmental toxins.** We live in a toxic world. Our outdoor world may be laced with pesticides and herbicides. Our homes tend to contain toxic household cleaning materials and furniture, rugs and construction materials that include formaldehyde and other hazardous chemicals. These toxins have far-reaching effects on all body systems, including the respiratory system, increasing the probability of airway dysfunction and aggravating allergies that further limit airway capacity.

» **Action: NO removing teeth for orthodontic treatment.** If the orthodontist wants to remove teeth, run away as fast as you can and take your child with you.

Pulling teeth causes the jaw to recede rather than grow wider. An orthodontist who is knowledgeable about opening airways will help to expand your child's palate. Orthodontic success does not consist merely of "proper" teeth alignment without spaces.

We believe basic criteria for orthodontic success should be:

- no clicking, popping or locking of jaws;
- no headache;

- a wide broad smile;
- a good profile;
- no snoring or noisy breathing.

We have seen too many patients whose airway and jaw problems began at the age they had orthodontic treatment. Typically, children come under the care of orthodontists in their tween years (the "between" years, typically between 8 and 12) when they get braces, and possibly even head gear. Part of the traditional orthodontic process may include pulling of teeth to make space for the crowded, crooked teeth (typically a result of longer, narrower jaws).

However, pulling teeth actually shrinks the palate and jaws over time and is therefore counterproductive. Even worse, headgear typically pulls the jaws back too far, exacerbating airway blockage.

We have found that children as young as 3 will respond well to a palate expander to widen the upper jaw so the top and bottom teeth fit together better with improved nasal breathing and more room for the tongue and lower jaw. Terms that might be used for such treatments include: rapid maxillary expansion, palatal expansion, functional orthodontics, and BioBloc orthotropics. This widening and forward movement of the jaws at a young age often reduces the need for later orthodontia, especially when hypotonia is also addressed through OMT.

Such patterns are apparent by age 3, but can even be diagnosed at birth. When it comes to using a palate expander, the earlier treatment begins for the child, the better. Orthodontic intervention to expand the palate at age 3, coupled with re-establishing nasal breathing, proper diet and improved sleep will redirect the child's growth onto the proper path.

» **Action: Sleep study.** If your child has sleep-disordered breathing, ADHD, bed-wetting, night terrors or colic, insist on a sleep study. If your child struggles in school, mouth-breathes, or is overweight and craves sugar, a formal evaluation of her sleep patterns will help uncover what forms of sleep-disordered breathing she may be experiencing, and how SDBs are affecting her sleep. Being proactive could save her health, and prevent her from having life-long struggles with learning, mental focus, anxiety and depression.

» **Action (the 13th - a baker's dozen, and a parent's bonus-brownie point for being a great mom or dad): Time and attention.** Children who grow up in homes with parents who read to them and who provide enriching experiences are protected against the impact of many developmental problems. The extra time and attention that parents offer not only creates new learning opportunities for children, but also stimulate new connections between brain cells, that this can help increase a child's natural curiosity and self-confidence.

Other simple parenting and environmental choices by parents can make a difference—even changing bed sheets more regularly. Dirty sheets can attract dust mites and other allergens, causing nasal swelling which can aggravate a child's breathing problems, especially while they sleep.

Parents and their Child's Interdisciplinary Team

We invite you to see yourself as the coach of your child's team of healthcare and education providers. Chances are, your child's teachers, pediatrician, and dentist still have no idea how important it is to be opening airways for children, nor are they likely to know how to do it.[16] Because the research is scattered across a wide variety of disciplines, many pediatricians, dentists and ENT specialists simply are not yet up-to-date on the importance of unobstructed breathing during sleep and the far-reaching effects of airway obstruction.

Please don't accept at face value the negative information you're told about treatments for teeth, mouths, jaws, airways, or tongues

---

16 Speaking at the AAPMD conference, spring 2014, in Chicago, Dr Stephen Sheldon, MD, Professor of Pediatrics, Northwestern University, Feinberg School of Medicine and Director of Sleep Medicine Center Lurie Children's Hospital of Chicago, pointed out that for years, *Nelson's Textbook of Pediatrics*, a 2,200-page volume, had only 19 paragraphs on sleep. The most recent addition, according to Dr Sheldon, has 2,500-2,600 pages, and only 12 pages on sleep.

by other health care providers if they are not educated about the importance of opening airways. If they cannot cite research studies that we have given you above, like the work of Dr Karen Bonuck or Dr David Gozal, and if they don't know about opening airways through orthotropics and palatal expansion, then they are not the experts for you and your child.

And as you will see later in the book, this applies to you as well, because adults can also be treated to open their airways.

Specifically, we urge you to reject negative answers for either your child or yourself such as these:

Sleep-Disordered Breathing (SDB) symptoms:

» Pay attention early to your child's breathing and sleep.
» Be vigilant.
» Snoring and mouth breathing are the most obvious early signs of trouble.
» Recognition of problems and early intervention can prevent lifelong health challenges.
» Be the coach for your child's health, and don't give up.

» "Your (or your child's) pain/ problem won't go away."
» "You don't need your tongue/ frenulum released."
» "You'll never get better."
» "ADHD is a disease; it never goes away."
» "That treatment (Biobloc, myofunctional therapy, frenulum release, dental appliances) won't help you or your child."
» "We'll just watch your tonsils." (Or your child's tonsils)
» "Your child's jaw is too narrow. We have to take out two or four permanent teeth."

The purpose of the information offered here is to empower you—as coach of your child's interdisciplinary team—to take charge of your child's healthcare, while potentially addressing learning issues and problem behaviors in a whole new way.

6

C H A P T E R

For Adults Who are Tired of Feeling Sick and Tired

Ellen was referred to my office for jaw clicking and locking, sinus pain, neck pain and fatigue. Her jaw had dropped back by over 7 mm, resulting in airway collapse and decreased facial support. After inserting a lower repositioning Airway Centric® appliance to bring the lower jaw forward with increased support and facial height, symptoms began to improve. During sleep we were able to keep Ellen's lower jaw forward with an upper anti retrusion Airway Centric® sleep appliance.

Ellen's before and after photos are astounding. Without any plastic surgery, she easily looks and feels 15 years younger. I am still amazed by the opening of her eyes and the changes in her neck. The coup de grâce is the final picture during orthodontic treatment. The common denominator in both these cases is the reduction in pain and fatigue with

LATERAL
BEFORE AND AFTER

Pre-Treatment
5-8-2012

Progress
1-8-2013

Peter, age 70, is a diabetic on medication who came to see Dr Howard Hindin for head pain and TMJ pain. Dr Hindin suspected sleep apnea, and recommended a sleep study, which found that Peter had moderate OSA.

Dr Hindin fitted Peter with an appliance which he wore just at night.

Between the appliance and "less carbs focus," Peter's "wake-up" sugar-level readings came down from a typical 180-200 to the low 120s.

After Peter's most recent appliance adjustment, his blood sugar level readings decreased to an average of 93-94. His worst sugar spikes at any time of the day are now below 140. His diabetes doctor is "very pleased" with Peter's results.

Peter also had nightmares with the sleep apnea, and now has fewer nightmares.

improved health and facial aesthetics by opening the airway.

Airway-Centered Disorder in Adults

Chris, age 37, is a young father with a new baby who came into Dr Gelb's office for help because of his sleep apnea. His AHI, or apnea-hypopnea index, was 39.5, which means that while sleeping, Chris had an apnea or hypopnea episode almost 40 times every hour. So, he was losing oxygen more than once every other minute all night long.

Chris told us, "I used to wake up gasping. I would fall asleep watching a game and wake up gasping." Chris snored, and had a narrow airway. After treatment by Dr Gelb, Chris reports that he "sleeps well" (despite the new baby!) and no longer feels as "drowsy" during the day.

Gasping for breath is only one of the adult symptoms of sleep-disordered breathing. If you find yourself clenching or grinding your teeth, your spouse pokes you at night to get you to turn over and stop snoring, your head is constantly thrust forward in front of your shoulders, or your tongue has scalloped edges, then you most likely have airway-centered disorder.

The brain's primary goal is ensuring survival, so breathing well is one of its top priorities. Think of it this way: we humans evolved to breathe through our mouths as well as our noses, because otherwise, a cold or allergy attack would literally kill us when it

Lauren – A Beautiful Life Transformation

When Lauren, age 52, first came to see Dr Howard Hindin, she was significantly overweight, felt and looked exhausted, suffered from sleep apnea, smoked, and didn't even want her picture taken. Even though she had received dental care all her life and had braces at age 11, no one had ever told her that her palate was too small (the size of a 6-year-old's palate) and not leaving enough room for her tongue.

Dr Hindin fitted Lauren with a palate expander, which they have used to increase her palatal width by ¼ inch over a period of 13 months.

As a result of using the appliance, Lauren now sleeps better. She no longer wakes up with OSA, and no longer talks in her sleep.

"My dreams are different, I wake up feeling refreshed."

After about 7 months with the appliance expanding her palate, Lauren

"Really started to shift."

What does she now experience? Lauren could hardly contain her excitement as she explained: "I'm brighter (mentally brighter, energetically brighter), more focused, I sleep better. I'm getting stronger and stronger. I smile differently. I look differently. What Paula [Fabbie, OMT] has done – I speak differently. When you're sleeping better, everything is better – your physical attitude, mental attitude, your energy – everything's better. No more suffering from depression, no medications for depression. My confidence has increased, I am presenting myself differently to the world."

On top of all these benefits from having her palate expanded in her fifties, Lauren has quit smoking and lost weight.

closes off the nasal passageways! So, when the nose is stuffed, the mouth becomes the crucial gateway.

However, mouth breathing is strictly the emergency mode. It's fairly common, but it is neither the normal nor healthy ideal. Mouth breathing, does not warm, filter, and humidify the air entering our bodies the way nasal breathing does. Mouth breathing also does not produce nitric oxide in the breath, as nasal breathing does.[1]

---

1 Kevin, Boyd, DDS, "Malocclusion – Risk Factor for Obstructive Sleep Apnea (OSA) in children: A Darwinian Perspective," presented at the American Academy of Physiological Medicine and Dentistry conference, April 25-26, 2014.

If you:

- » Wake up feeling tired and often have headaches
- » Snore, or even wake up gasping for breath in the middle of the night
- » Clench or grind your teeth at night
- » Wake up frequently at night to use the bathroom
- » Have diabetes, high blood pressure, or cardiovascular disease
- » Are overweight or obese
- » Crave sugar, junk food, or caffeine
- » Often feel sleepy during the day or have trouble staying awake while driving
- » Have difficulty concentrating or adult onset attention deficit hyperactivity disorder
- » Have difficulties with allergies, sinus problems, or ear infections
- » Feel as though you are often in a mental fog
- » Feel energetically drained and always "too tired to exercise"

.... Then you most likely don't get enough sleep, or you have an airway issue that keeps you from sleeping deeply and restfully.

Yet many people are mouth-breathers, some consistently, others occasionally. If you think you are not a mouth-breather, try reading each word of this paragraph out loud, one word at a time, emphasizing each word, and breathing in through your nose after each word. If this is difficult for you to do, chances are that you are a partial mouth-breather, even if only while talking (or perhaps singing).

We can work to prevent sleep-disordered breathing and ACD-related issues early in life or at any point along the way. It's never too late to improve your breathing and your health, no matter how old you are. Peter, age 70, whose story is above, is only one of many older patients whom we have helped with their sleep and breathing, so that they could stop feeling sick and tired all the time. In Lauren's story, you can see that we used an orthopedic device to expand the palate of a fifty-something!

With the Airway Centric® Model, significant improvements in health can be made as various medical professionals—from ENT specialists and allergists, to dentists, orthodontists and orofacial myofunctional therapists (OMTs), occupational therapists (OTs), speech language pathologists (SLPs), physical therapists, and chiropractors—all collaborate as an interdisciplinary team. The necessary practitioners develop, maintain and restore the airway, and they teach proper breathing techniques. This approach enhances facial proportions at any age.

Clues to Watch For

Sometimes SDB breathing issues can look like another problem, so we look for other clues. Many of us visit the dentist because of teeth grinding, TMJ pain, or headaches. Many of us visit the neurologist for help with restless legs, or maybe visit an internist for sleeping pills, or a chiropractor because of back pain. Rarely do these medical specialists connect with each other, look at these issues holistically, and relate them back to an airway problem. And yet, many of the conditions can be related directly to a blocked airway.

We had one patient who complained of restless leg syndrome (RLS). She was taking Valium and Librium to help calm her body and control the shaking. She had low iron levels as well. But we determined that her problem was not neurological, nor was it related to anemia, even though RLS has been linked to anemia. Our patient was tossing and turning all night because she was struggling for air. Her first clue: waking up to a wrinkled bed with twisted blankets and sheets. People who sleep deeply often wake up in a bed that almost looks like it is still made.

Many people believe the need to urinate wakes them up. Yet we find that when an airway opens, Mother Nature's midnight wakeup calls abruptly stop because deep sleep relaxes your body and enables you to sleep through the night. In fact, researchers in Israel found an association between nighttime awakening to urinate (nocturia) in men with benign prostate enlargement and symptoms of obstructive sleep apnea. Their statistical results were so strong, they concluded that, even with benign prostate enlargement, these men, aged 55-75, may be awakening because of sleep apnea episodes, and only then feeling the urge to urinate.[2]

Adults Need Adequate Sleep

Experts recommend seven to nine hours of sleep for adults, but, hectic schedules, electronic media, work demands and family pressures prevent most American adults from getting that much. The Centers for Disease Control and Prevention tells us that, on average, 30% of American adults who work get six hours of sleep or less each night.[3]

If you are one of the millions of adults with sleep-disordered breathing, even if you do spend the recommended seven to nine hours in bed, you still might feel drowsy throughout the day, not energetic enough to accomplish tasks, and never wide awake. No matter how much coffee you drink in the morning, no matter how many cookies and candies you eat during the day, no amount of sugar and caffeine can give you enough energy to get everything done. And that wouldn't be good for your overall health.

If you have an obstructed airway and sleep-related issues, you're probably not getting enough sleep. Here's a strong indicator that can help you on your way to a diagnosis: even after eight or more hours in bed, you feel groggy and have difficulty getting out of bed in the morning.

The Vicious Cycle

When airway obstruction prevents you from getting deep restful sleep, a vicious cycle begins. Suppose you get to bed at 10 p.m., drift off to sleep in just a few minutes, only to find yourself wide awake at 2 a.m., unable to go back to sleep and eventually drifting

2 Tandeter, Howard, MD, et al, "Nocturic Episodes in Patients with Benign Prostatic Enlargement May Suggest the Presence of Obstructive Sleep Apnea," *Journal of the American Board of Family Medicine*, March-April 2011, Volume 24, Number 2, 146-151. http://www.jabfm.org/content/24/2/146.short

3 "Short Sleep Duration Among Workers — United States, 2010," *Morbidity and Mortality Weekly Report (MMWR)* April 27, 2012 / 61(16); 281-285. http://www.cdc.gov/mmwr/preview/mmwrhtml/mm6116a2.htm?s_cid=mm6116a2_w

back off just before the alarm sounds. Yes, you've been in bed for eight hours, but you've really only gotten four or five hours of sleep, and even that was interrupted.

Chances are—unless you're under the influence of the hormonal fluctuations of menopause or are suffering from severe anxiety— that your 2 a.m. wake up call was caused by sleep apnea or some type of airway obstruction (and not because you needed a trip to the bathroom). When you have a sleep apnea episode, you literally stop breathing. So, you have probably awakened coughing or gasping for air with your heart pounding. When you stop breathing, as can happen dozens of times an hour with sleep apnea, your body engages in the stress response, sometimes called the fight-flight-or-freeze response. Adrenaline pumps through your system, supercharging your mind so it can make instant decisions, and through your muscles so you can run or fight for your life.

You awaken in the darkness, perhaps even unaware that you had stopped breathing. But those brain chemicals that flooded your body won't let your body or mind forget. That's why you're staring at the ceiling as the clock ticks away the hours.

The energetic expenditure of that adrenaline rush gobbles up glucose from your system, so your blood sugar drops. Some people with sleep disturbances like this even find themselves eating in the middle of the night.

Maybe you finally drift back off to sleep for an hour or two before the alarm goes off and you drag your weary, sleep-deprived self out of bed, hardly in shape to start a new day.

What's the first thing you reach for (hopefully after your toothbrush)? It's probably a cup of coffee. Caffeine is a temporary "fix" for your energy crisis, but it's only temporary.

Maybe you eat some breakfast. A muffin to go with your sugary coffee drink? Does that sound familiar? Or maybe you opt out of breakfast, too tired and rushed to get to work and the kids off to school that your can't even think about food.

By 10 a.m., you're famished and your energy level is dropping, probably just before that big meeting where you have to make a presentation. So you grab a quick snack, maybe something out of the vending machine or you raid that bag of cookies in your bottom drawer or the donuts your helpful co-workers left in the break room.

At noon, you go out to lunch with co-workers, full of good intention that you'll order a salad, but that burger and fries looks so good...

By 4 p.m., you can barely stay awake. An energy fix of a double espresso and a biscotti or another muffin helps you get through that last grueling hour.

As you leave work, you are thinking: "a late afternoon workout? Are you kidding?" You have no energy for exercise. Then it's time to battle traffic on the way home, and fight the urge to yell at the kids while you're wondering what to fix for dinner.

Instead of a relaxing evening, you're plagued with forgotten permission slips, unfolded laundry, a phone call from your mother and a few urgent e-mails you must return.

At 9 p.m., you have a sudden craving for ice cream. You deserve a reward, don't you?

Suddenly it's 10 p.m. and you fall into bed, exhausted beyond all imagination, only to start the whole process over again.

Does any of this sound familiar?

It's a sadly typical narration of modern life for so many of us. It's just life and stress, you answer. We suggest that it's not just stress—it's a pattern you can break if you open your airway.

A Little Sleep Science

Sleep fragmentation occurs with sleep-disordered breathing. Sleep fragmentation can be measured a number of ways; one commonly-agreed on practice is by measuring EEG changes that last at least three seconds. Commonly, what we refer to as sleep fragmentation is the interruption of deep, slow wave sleep, as shown by EEG patterns which indicate that the sleeper has gone into a lighter stage of sleep. However, some degree of interference with sleep can occur without necessarily causing changes in EEG patterns, for instance, when significant changes in blood pressure or heart rate occur without changing EEG patterns. So, sleep fragmentation ranges from significant cardiovascular changes to EEG arousals that lighten the stage of sleep, to full awakening.[4]

Much of the sleep fragmentation of sleep-disordered breathing stems from respiratory effort-related arousals (RERAs). RERAs are events in which the sleeper has difficulty breathing, as measured by changes in upper airway pressure, that lead to some degree of arousal, which is often measured by changes in EEG showing that the stage of deep sleep ended and a lighter stage of sleep was entered. RERAs reflect a limitation on the amount of air flow during each breath. These limitations do not entail either apneas or hypopneas. Researchers at the New York University School of Medicine found that a non-invasive technique, the nasal cannula/ pressure transducer, can be used to detect flow limitations resulting from pressure changes in the upper airway.[5]

Whether from apneas, hypopneas, or RERAs, the resulting sleep fragmentation interrupts the deep Stage 3 and 4 delta sleep cycles as well as REM sleep, preventing your brain and body from experiencing physiologically refreshing sleep. Researchers have coined the term: "sleep continuity hypothesis" to express the fact that much research suggests that when sleep fragmentation interrupts the restorative process of a deep stage of

If we have sleep apnea:

Subconsciously, the brain puts itself on high alert before bedtime, knowing that the life-giving oxygen will be compromised by a blocked airway as soon as we lie down to sleep.

The result: we subconsciously fear and avoid going to sleep. This physiologically-based, blocked airway-driven resistance to going to sleep constitutes a greatly-overlooked root cause of much of adult insomnia.

---

4 Stepanski, Edward J, "The Effect of Sleep Fragmentation on Daytime Function," *Sleep*, Vol. 25, No. 3, 2002, 268-276. http://www.journalsleep. org/articles/250302.pdf

5 Ayappa, Indu, PhD, et al, "Non-invasive Detection of Respiratory Effort-Related Arousals (RERAs) by a Nasal Cannula/Pressure Transducer System," *Sleep*, Vol. 23, No 6, 2000, 763-771. http://www.journalsleep.org/Articles/230605.pdf

sleep, the benefits of that restorative cycle are lost.[6] (See the sleep chart on page 52.)

High Adrenaline, SDBs, and Insomnia

People who have an airway problem (ACD) express it at night as sleep-disordered breathing (SDBs). Because the brain recognizes that oxygen deficiency, people with ACD are in a constant state of high adrenaline. They go-go-go and then they crash. It is as if they are a car with only an on-off switch, but no accelerator and no brakes: it's all or nothing.

When a person's body is tired and running on adrenaline, it's not surprising that he or she become anxious, irritable and exhausted at the same time. That's certainly not a good recipe for a peaceful night's sleep, so the vicious cycle repeats night after night.

When children are overtired, their extreme fatigue often looks like hyperactivity. That hidden fatigue is why something like Ritalin—a form of speed—calms them down. But in adults—even in the late teens—lack of sleep usually looks like overall fatigue and a lack of energy. Sometimes, though, sleep deprivation in adults can also resemble hyperactivity, so that adults find themselves consciously or even sub-consciously doing whatever it takes to keep that adrenaline rush. The imbalance of hormones and the brain's defense against not having enough oxygen all night can create anxiety, and the need to keep going despite fatigue can trigger that physiological anxiety to remain along with the adrenaline rush.

We know that if children have open airways, they are more likely to get deeper sleep and are more agreeable about going to bed. But if the airway is compromised even slightly, they are less likely to want to sleep, perhaps instinctively fearing those breathing-related abrupt wake-ups.

As adults, we react in much the same way. Subconsciously, the brain puts itself on high alert before bedtime, knowing that the life-giving oxygen will be compromised by a blocked airway as soon as we lie down to sleep. The result: we subconsciously fear and avoid going to sleep. This physiologically-based, blocked air-

---

6 Stepanski, Edward.

way-driven resistance to sleeping constitutes a greatly-overlooked root cause of much of adult insomnia.

Like little kids who have tantrums at bedtime and fight sleep, we adults have our own form of bedtime "tantrums," or efforts to cope, knowing on an instinctive level that sleep is dangerous. For adults, this bedtime resistance may take the form of anxiety, including anxiety about insomnia, as well as a subconscious fear of falling asleep.

If you stay up late watching television, and then you eventually fall asleep on the couch thinking that boring television show is the sleep inducer, you may have SDB.

People with compromised airways are sleep deprived, fatigued and exhausted. It is not the TV show that bores them to sleep. They find it easy to fall asleep sitting up because their tongues aren't as far back in their mouths, so the airway is open. They fall asleep on the couch, but when they awaken and go up to bed they cannot get back to sleep. As soon as they lie down, their brains and bodies go on alert: "Breathing will be difficult! It is too dangerous to lie down! Stay awake!" They become flush with adrenaline, too tense to sleep in bed.

> **People find it easy** to fall asleep sitting up because their tongues aren't as far back in their mouths, so the airway is open. As soon as they lie down, their brains and bodies go on alert: "Breathing will be difficult! It is too dangerous to lie down! Stay awake!" They become flush with adrenaline, too tense to sleep in bed.

Sleepiness vs Fatigue

Pain and fatigue are two of the biggest reasons for doctor visits. We all understand pain, but fatigue seems vague and difficult to explain. Essentially, fatigue doesn't allow us to get things done. When we feel chronically fatigued, we can't function, we don't have optimal energy for relationships, and we can't sustain our job performance. When we feel fatigued day after day, somehow we just muddle on.

You can be fatigued without being sleepy the way you can be "not sick," but that doesn't mean you are well. Being fatigued means feeling tired as you go about your day. You feel exhausted, with low energy and lack of concentration. It seems you can't accomplish anything.

Chronic fatigue can be connected to a host of other health problems—from depression to headaches to muscle aches to cardiac problems. Perhaps you're already guessing what we'll say next: a blocked airway can lie at the root of all of those problems, including the underlying chronic fatigue.

Fatigue is different than sleepiness. Sleepy people can get a lot done. Fatigued people cannot. And for fatigued people, sleep doesn't help. It doesn't refresh the body or mind.

Sleepiness is a state that invites sleep. Sleepiness means you have the readiness to fall asleep. Simply put, you can't keep your eyes open.

Unfortunately, people with sleep apnea often do not fully realize how sleepy they are. One study found that patients with obstructive sleep apnea significantly underestimated their own sleepiness until after they had received treatment.[7] This inability to discern their sleepiness may occur because of the loss of executive functions such as judgment due to the negative impact of SDBs on the prefrontal cortex.[8]

As doctors who look at airways, we are concerned about sleepiness and fatigue. We know the importance of treating SDBs because we know what a devastating impact they can have on your life.

For some patients, we recommend a Multiple Sleep Latency Test, which aims to discover how readily he or she can fall asleep. At a sleep clinic, the patient is given four or five chances to take a 20-minute nap over a two-hour period. Brain waves (EEG), muscle

---

7 Guimaraes, C. Martins, M.V., Rodrigues, L., Texixeira, F., and Moutinho Dos Santos, J., "Epworth Sleepiness Scale in Obstructive Sleep Apnea Syndrome – an Underestimated Subjective Scale," *Portuguese Journal of Pulmonology*, 2012 Nov; 18(6): 267-271, as cited in: B*est of Sleep Medicine* 2013, Teofilo Lee-Chiong, 2014, p. 99.

8 Magdalena Nowak, MD; Johannes Kornhuber, MD; Robert Meyrer, MD, "Daytime Impairment and Neurodegeneration in OSAS," *Sleep*, Vol. 29, No. 12, 2006, 1521-1530. http://www.journalsleep.org/Articles/291201.pdf

activity, and eye movements are checked and recorded. This information helps doctors determine the type of sleep interruption and what can be done with it.

The Full Body Picture: Fat, Sick, and Tired

As a result of the cascade of health challenges that SDBs set in motion, our bodies get out-of-balance. Our health and our sense of well-being diminish. Sleep-disordered breathing creates systemic problems for the entire body—impacting mental health as well as physical health. As researchers in Finland best expressed it: "Sleep-disordered breathing (SDB) is not only a problem of the upper airway *but is a systemic condition* with endocrine and metabolic interactions."[9] (Italics added)

The interaction of sleep-disordered breathing with hormone levels causes SDBs to go hand-in-hand with obesity, fatigue, and diabetes, i.e., SDBs contribute to obesity, diabetes, and fatigue, and vice versa.

For example, researchers have found that reduced amounts of sleep cause decreased levels of leptin, a hormone which "tells the brain enough food has been consumed,"[10] thereby causing satiety, the feeling of fullness. So, when we don't get enough sleep, we lack sufficient amounts of the chemical which tells our stomachs we have had enough to eat, and our judgment of portion size is impaired, which often induces overeating.

In addition, sleep reduction increases the levels of grehlin, a hormone that stimulates appetite.[11] This means that when we don't sleep long enough, we literally have a chemical in our bodies signaling us to eat more. In other words, the two brain chemicals which lead us either to feel full or to crave food get completely reversed when we don't get enough sleep or don't sleep well. This

---

9 Saaresranta, T., and O Polo. "Sleep-disordered breathing and hormones," *European Respiratory Journal*, July 1, 2003. Vol. 22 No. 1, 161-172. http://erj.ersjournals.com/content/22/1/161.full

10 Brody, Jane, E., "Cheating Ourselves of Sleep," *The New York Times*, June 17, 2013. http://well.blogs.nytimes.com/2013/06/17/cheating-our-selves-of-sleep/

11 Ibid.

chemical imbalance results in us craving food, especially sugary foods and junk food.

A fascinating study from the University of California at Berkeley showed that young adults who were not allowed to sleep were more likely to reach for donuts and pizza than healthier foods. The lack of sleep suppressed the prefrontal cortex, which is responsible for complex decision-making, judgment, and stimulating the reward-seeking part of the brain.[12] While the study does not discuss this, the researchers were looking at brain stimulation rather than hormonal effects; leptin and grehlin receptor cells are located in the hypothalamus, not the prefrontal cortex.

While many of these studies looked solely at shorter durations of sleep, other studies found similar results in terms of changes in brain chemistry from sleep-disordered breathing.[13] Many of the physiological changes that occur from sleeping fewer hours also happen when our sleep is disturbed due to obstructive sleep apnea, because sleep apnea disrupts both deep (slow-wave) sleep and REM sleep.[14] Over the years, many studies have found similar effects of both short duration of sleep and fragmented sleep, such as occurs with obstructive sleep apnea.[15]

Numerous studies show that those who sleep fewer hours tend to weigh more than those who get sufficient sleep.[16] Research also

---

12 Anwar, Yasmin, "Sleep deprivation linked to junk food cravings," Berkeley Media Relations, August 6, 2013. http://newscenter.berkeley.edu/2013/08/06/poor-sleep-junk-food/

13 See, for instance, Saaresranta and Polo above.

14 Carskadon, M.A., & Dement, W.C. (2011). "Monitoring and staging human sleep." In M.H. Kryger, T. Roth, & W.C. Dement (Eds.), *Principles and Practice of Sleep Medicine*, 5th edition, (pp 16-26). St. Louis: Elsevier Saunders. http://apsychoserver.psych.arizona.edu/jjbareprints/psyc501a/readings/Carskadon%20Dement%202011.pdf

15 Stepanski, Edward J. The studies he reviewed mostly linked sleep fragmentation with the problems associated with excessive daytime sleepiness, not yet looking at the underlying causes of those problems.

16 Buxton, Orfeu M, et al, "Association of Sleep Adequacy With More Healthful Food Choices and Positive Workplace Experiences Among Motor Freight Workers," *American Journal of Public Health*, 2009 November; 99(Suppl 3): S636–S643. http://www.ncbi.nlm.nih.gov/pmc/

shows us that being overweight affects sleep cycles and increases the risk of sleep apnea. Sleep quality declines, hormone levels regulating appetite and cravings are disrupted, and food cravings increase, resulting in more weight gain and even less restful sleep. Together, these issues conspire to create a downward spiral that can—and often does—lead to diabetes, heart disease and certain types of cancer.

One study found that 82% of diabetics have obstructive sleep apnea. These researchers also found that "diabetics had almost double the risk of carbohydrate craving of non-diabetics." In addition, the study showed that patients with obstructive sleep apnea "were almost twice as likely to have high carbohydrate craving as patients without sleep apnea."[17]

Thus, it seems logical to consider short sleep duration along with sleep apnea and other forms of SDBs a primary cause of obesity.

Among the 69.2% of American adults who are overweight, there are higher rates of diabetes, cardiovascular disease, and other health-related issues. It's well past time to make efforts to stem this tide of "metabolic syndrome."

This syndrome refers to the body having an increased risk for a triad of unhealthiness: obesity, diabetes, and cardiovascular disease. Study after study shows the link between diabetes and sleep-disordered breathing, in part because increased BMI (body mass index, a measure of how much fat a person has) is a main risk factor for snoring and sleep apnea.[18]

---

articles/PMC2774168/. See also: Brody, Jane E., "Cheating Ourselves of Sleep," *The New York Times Blog*, June 17, 2013. http://well.blogs.nytimes.com/2013/06/17/cheating-ourselves-of-sleep/

17 Sleep and Wellness Medical Associates, LLC of New Jersey. Research results provided to Medical Express News by the American Academy of Sleep Medicine and presented at the 2012 Sleep conference. http://medicalxpress.com/news/2012-06-apnea-linked-carbohydrate-craving-diabetics.html

18 AlDabal, Laila, and Ahmed S. Bahammam, "Metabolic, Endocrine, and Immune Consequences of Sleep Deprivation," *The Open Respiratory Medicine Journal,* 2011; 5:31-43. Published online June 23, 2011. http://www.ncbi.nlm.nih.gov/pmc/articles/PMC3132857/

Studies also show that sleep-disordered breathing leads to glucose intolerance and alters the body's ability to process glucose.[19] One study prevented healthy young men from getting more than four hours of sleep for just six nights in a row, and found that they "ended up with insulin and blood sugar levels like those of people deemed pre-diabetic."[20]

So, if you are overweight and have difficulty sleeping, your risk of becoming diabetic is high. We recommend that you have a sleep study to address any sleep-disordered breathing that may be contributing to you developing "metabolic syndrome." Your health—even your life—may depend on it.

Adults need at least 22-24% of their sleep to be composed of deep, delta wave, or slow wave sleep. Among the important functions of deep stage sleep in adults is the release of human growth hormone, which repairs and maintains healthy muscles, including the heart. Growth hormone also maintains a healthy metabolism, providing energy for the day ahead. Importantly, growth hormone helps maintain healthy cholesterol balances and bone density. It also regulates fat deposits, maintains lean muscle mass, and promotes brain health.[21]

Sleep apnea reduces slow wave sleep, so it also reduces the output of growth hormone. The reduced oxygenation of the blood that can occur with sleep apnea (hypoxemia) can also reduce the body's tendency to release growth hormone. Even obesity, which often goes hand-in-hand with sleep apnea, can reduce the release of growth hormone.[22] Put together, sleep-disordered breathing and obesity can significantly alter hormone levels.

One of the reasons you may feel sick and tired is that sleep-disordered breathing, particularly obstructive sleep apnea (OSA), affects cardiovascular health. Notably, one study of OSA in men over a 10-year period found that those with untreated, severe ob-

---

19 Ibid.

20 Brody, Jane E.

21 http://www.cedars-sinai.edu/Patients/Health-Conditions/
Adult-Growth-Hormone-Deficiency.aspx and http://www.gene.com/
patients/disease-education/understanding-human-growth-hormone

22 Saaresranta, T., et al.

structive sleep apnea had significantly higher rates of cardiovascular disease, with both fatal and non-fatal cardiovascular events, when compared to healthy men, men who simply snored, and men with mild to moderate sleep apnea. This same study found that men with OSA who received CPAP treatment had a significantly lowered risk of cardiovascular disease compared with men with untreated OSA.[23]

Several physiological processes may contribute to cardiovascular disease because of sleep-disordered breathing, particularly OSA. First, there is the reduction of oxygen and the increase of carbon dioxide, a combo that's stressing the cells of both brain and body. This starts that cascade of stress hormone responses, especially adrenaline, but also includes increased cortisol spikes during apneic events.[24] Elevated cortisol levels due to stress have been linked to elevated cardiovascular risks.[25]

Sleep apnea has been strongly linked to elevated blood pressure, as well as increased heart rate, during episodes of apnea.[26,27] People with OSA have also been found to have elevated

23 Marin, JM, et al, "Long-term cardiovascular outcomes in men with obstructive sleep apnoea-hypopnoea with or without treatment with continuous positive airway pressure: an observational study," *Lancet*, 2005 Mar 19-25; 365(9464):1046-53. http://www.ncbi.nlm.nih.gov/pubmed/15781100

24 Karon, Amy, "Nocturnal Cortisol Levels Predicted Neurocognitive Impairment in Sleep Apnea," *Clinical Psychiatry News Digital Network*, May 1, 2014, Clinical Psychiatry News. http://www.clinicalpsychiatrynews.com/home/article/nocturnal-cortisol-levels-predicted-neurocognitive-impairment-in-sleep-apnea/b80679e1cb98613d0c084d56bcdb926b.html

25 Boyles, Salynn, "Stress Hormone Predicts Heart Death: High Cortisol Levels Raise Risk of Heart Disease, Stroke 5-Fold," *WebMD Health News* Sept. 9, 2010. http://www.webmd.com/heart-disease/news/20100909/stress-hormone-predicts-heart-death

26 Peters, Brandon, M.D., "Sleep Apnea and the Risks to Heart Health: Untreated OSA May Lead to High Blood Pressure, Diabetes, and Heart Attacks," March 20, 2014. *About.com*: http://sleepdisorders.about.com/od/sleepandgeneralhealth/fl/Sleep-Apnea-and-the-Risks-to-Heart-Health.htm

27 Mitchell Miglis, M.D., "What Untreated Sleep Apnea Means for Your Blood Pressure," Stanford Center for Sleep Sciences and Medicine, *Huffpost Healthy Living*, Posted: 07/25/2013 8:16 am. http://www.huffing-

daytime levels of both adrenaline and blood pressure.[28] Moreover, inadequate sleep has been linked to calcification of the arteries.[29] So, a variety of factors associated with sleep apnea contribute to a significantly-elevated risk of cardiovascular disease.

Inflammation is another physiological process that is worsened by sleep-disordered breathing. Increased inflammatory compounds, including c-reactive proteins and cytokines, contribute to the progression of cardiovascular disease in people with OSA.[30] One study found that OSA patients had increased levels of HDL cholesterol correlated with increases in the severity of their AHI index, but when they were treated with CPAP machines, their serum cholesterol levels improved significantly.[31]

> **Obstructive sleep apnea** increases the likelihood of cardiovascular disease, diabetes, obesity, acid reflux, and even fatal cancer.

The bottom line: obstructive sleep apnea significantly increases your risk of having a fatal stroke or heart attack. If that isn't enough bad news, sleep-disordered breathing also negatively affects your immune system, possibly contributing to that feeling of being sick and tired of being sick and tired. According to Dr Deepak Shrivastava of the University of California's Davis School of Medicine, OSA

---

tonpost.com/stanford-center-for-sleep-sciences-and-medicine/connection-between-sleep-apnea-and-high-blood-pressure_b_3633005.html

28 Ibid.

29 Brody, Jane E.

30 Shrivastava, Deepak, MD, "Impact of Sleep Disordered Breathing on Upper Airway Anatomy and Physiology," presented to the American Academy of Physiological Medicine and Dentistry, April 2014. http://aapmd.org/ See also: Ryan, Silke, et al, "Selective Activation of Inflammatory Pathways by Intermittent Hypoxia in Obstructive Sleep Apnea Syndrome," *Circulation, American Heart Association Journals*, http://circ.ahajournals.org/content/112/17/2660.full

31 Borgel, J., et al, Obstructive Sleep Apnoea and Its Therapy Influence High-Density Lipoprotein Cholesterol Serum Levels," *European Respiratory Journal*, 2006, 27: 121-127. http://erj.ersjournals.com/content/27/1/121.full.pdf

decreases the number of lymphocytes, and thus reduces the effectiveness of the immune system.[32]

During sleep, the production and levels of T-cells and interleukin-12 are enhanced, whereas sleep deprivation has the reverse influence.[33] Sleep deprivation has been found to increase levels of B cells, which not only contribute to the body's defense system, but which also increase both allergies and asthma.[34]

Dr Steven Park, MD, author of *Sleep, Interrupted*, argues: "By definition, if you have a sleep-breathing problem, your immune system is overly active. And so is your nervous system. This is why your body over-reacts to weather changes, certain foods, emotions, pollens, chemicals, and even certain sounds."

He also points out: "most cases of sore or scratchy throat isn't really from the viral infection—it's from your stomach juices, which includes bile, digestive enzymes, acid, and bacteria."[35] Sleep-disordered breathing can cause stomach acid to rise into the throat. The collapse of the airway results in a narrowing of the upper airway passages, which in turn creates a negative pressure in the throat, causing the stomach contents literally to be sucked up into the throat while sleeping. This can result in GERD (gastroesophageal reflux disease or acid reflux).[36] The drawing of stomach acid into the throat can also result in that nagging soreness in the back of the throat that we often associate with post-nasal drip, along with the

---

32 See Shrivastava, above.

33 Besedovsky, Luciana, et al. "Sleep and Immune Function," Published online: 10 November 2011 with open access at Springerlink.com

34 University of Helsinki, "New links between sleep deprivation, immune system discovered," October 23, 2013, *Science Daily* http://www.science-daily.com/releases/2013/10/131023183908.htm

35 http://doctorstevenpark.com/colds-viruses-and-sleep-apnea. See also his book: *Sleep, Interrupted: A physician reveals the #1 reason why so many of us are sick and tired.* Steven Y. Park, MD, (Jodev Press: New York), 2008.

36 Vann, Madeline, MPH, 11 Health Risks of Snoring, *Everyday Health*, March 24, 2014. http://www.everydayhealth.com/news/eleven-health-risks-snoring/?xid=aol_eh-sleep_1_20140324_&aolcat=AJA&ncid=webmail30%20GERD

post-nasal drip and continuous need to "clear the throat."[37] In fact, researchers at Duke University found that treating patients who have both sleep apnea and GERD with a CPAP machine significantly reduced their nighttime acid reflux.[38]

Cancer and Sleep-Disordered Breathing

Researchers in Sydney, Australia followed patients with sleep apnea along with those without sleep apnea for 20 years, and found that the people with sleep apnea had a 3.4% higher rate of death from cancer.[39] Other researchers found that sleep apnea increases the likelihood of cancer due to the lack of oxygen (hypoxia) the body experiences during sleep apnea and hypopnea episodes.[40]

Researcher David Gozal of the University of Chicago found that fragmented sleep can induce the immune system to spur tumors to become more aggressive.[41] Gozal isolated the immune system chemical responsible for the aggressive tumors, a tumor-associated macrophage known as TLR4, noting that this increases the likelihood of treating the cancer effectively.

---

37 Gaynor, EB, "Otolaryngologic manifestations of gastroesophageal reflux," *The American Journal of Gastroenterology, 1991, 86 (7), 801-808. http://europepmc.org/abstract/MED/2058616*

38 Green, Bryan T., et al, "Marked Improvement in Nocturnal Gastroesophageal Reflux in a Large Cohort of Patients with Obstructive Sleep Apnea Treated with Continuous Positive Airway Pressure," *JAMA Internal Medicine*, January 2003, 163(1):41-45. http://archinte.jamanetwork.com/article.aspx?articleid=214918

39 Phend, Crystal, "Sleep Apnea Linked to Cancer," *Medpage Today,* April 15, 2014. http://www.medpagetoday.com/PrimaryCare/SleepDisorders/45272

40 Campos-Rodriguez, F., et al, "Association between obstructive sleep apnea and cancer incidence in a large multicenter Spanish cohort," *American Journal of Respiratory and Critical Care Medicine*, 2013 Jan 1; 187(1):99-105.

41 Easton, John, "Fragmented sleep accelerates cancer growth," *University of Chicago News*, January 27, 2014. http://news.uchicago.edu/article/2014/01/27/fragmented-sleep-accelerates-cancer-growth

Now, if all that science hasn't put you to sleep, it has inspired you to treat your sleep apnea or other form of sleep-disordered breathing so that you can wake up feeling refreshed, have sufficient energy for your day, lower your risk of cancer, diabetes, and heart disease, lose weight, and enjoy better health.

Behavior, Epigenetics, and Chemistry – It's Not Your Fault!

Patty arrived in our office complaining of jaw pain. Dressed in a sweat suit, she was fresh from her daily workout. In her late forties, Patty declared to us that she was "really focused" on staying fit.

Patty had a history of jaw pain and clicking since her teenage years. She had been diagnosed with temporomandibular joint disorder or TMJ nearly 20 years before. She told us her health is good, but now that she has entered menopause, her sleep is poor and in spite of all her best efforts, she continues to put on weight in all the wrong places.

She starts every day with the motivation to eat good food, sensible portions and avoid sugar and junk food. Every day something happens and she is snacking and craving more sugary foods. She told us she is always tired and she forces herself to exercise because she fears she will "be a blimp" if she stops working out.

"I have no willpower," she said. Her husband and friends were tired of hearing her complain of tiredness and weight problems. "My husband told me that if I really wanted to lose weight I would stop talking about it and do something," she confided in us.

Although Patty was in our office for a TMJ problem, her story about her battle with weight was an important element that helped us find the right diagnosis and treatment.

After a comprehensive TMJ exam with images provided by a CBCT (cone beam computed tomography) and MRI, it was determined that Patty had a dislocated disc in her jaw joint. But with her history, we suspected she also had an airway problem. The CBCT showed a diminished airway space, so a sleep study was ordered. The results: Patty had mild sleep apnea.

Although her case was mild, it appeared that Patty's system was working hard at night (and during the day, too) to maintain her airway. Her crowded and narrow dental arches had never been treated when she was a child, so she had been living with poor posture, clenching, bruxism and muscle tightness in an effort to maintain an adequate airway.

Patty's TMJ problem was treated with a TMJ/sleep appliance. She was referred to an endocrinologist and nutritionist. Today, Patty is doing much better. Her sleep has improved; she has more energy in the mornings; she eats a healthier breakfast making sure she has protein and fiber. She now finds it is easier to get to the gym and she has lost 12 pounds.

Most of all, she feels better about herself. With her understanding of how the triad airway/sleep, nutrition, and exercise can cause either a lifetime of health problems or wellness, she no longer feels defective and weak-willed. She feels empowered to take charge of her own health.

Now Patty is even considering orthodontic treatment to correct the crowded, narrow arches. She knows it will help her breathe better and now that she feels better, why not have a broader, brighter, more beautiful smile?

If you are like Patty, you may be blaming yourself for eating junk food and gaining weight, but when you have an airway issue, the chemistry of your brain and body are clearly changed, and may continue to change and worsen the longer your airway issue remains untreated. While you may find yourself succumbing to sugar cravings, we would like to emphasize that it's not a matter of blaming yourself for lack of willpower. Your brain and body chemistry may be making it nearly impossible for you to resist.

Over time, both age and obesity can significantly diminish the sensitivity of the leptin receptors in the brain.[42] Reversing that damage then becomes increasingly difficult, further reducing the capability to feel full.

---

42 You, Jia, et al, "Signaling through Tyr[985] of Leptin Receptor as an Age/Diet-Dependent Switch in the Regulation of Energy Balance," *Molecular and Cellular Biology,* Apr 2010; 30(7): 1650–1659. This study shows that increased age diminishes leptin sensitivity in mice.

Dr Robert Lustig, author of *Fat Chance: Beating the Odds Against Sugar, Processed Food, Obesity, and Disease*, points out that this inability to be responsive to leptin is the cause of obesity, meaning that obesity is really a result of brain and hormonal chemistry gone awry. It's very difficult to change these imbalances by dieting and that's why diets don't work in the long run.

Dr Lustig showed that when we eat sugar, our insulin level rises; this prompts increased insulin resistance, which then triggers resistance to leptin as well. Because of our brain's resistance to leptin, we literally don't feel full, and we crave more food. Given that our society surrounds us with sugary food options that were not available to our ancestors, it is no wonder that we find ourselves eating more sugar than we need. This standard diet leads to our brains telling us to keep eating. Dr Lustig stresses that it is not our will-power that is lacking, but our brain's chemical balance that is off.[43]

Then there's the theory that when you diet, your metabolism changes so you can survive on less food. Researchers at the University of Washington found that dieting increases levels of grehlin, the hunger hormone, in the body, leading to that vicious cycle of weight gain after dieting and weight loss.[44]

The hormones and chemical balance of our bodies are definitely influenced by epigenetic effects. Epigenetics is the new science that shows how profoundly our environment and lifestyle choices can affect our genetic structure and our lifelong health. Epigenetics, in this case, shows us that we can use our lifestyle choices to "turn on" the genetic structures that help overcome metabolic and brain chemistry imbalances and keep weight at appropriate levels.

---

43 Atkinson, Louise, "The REAL Reason You Eat too Much: New Theory Could Revolutionize the Way We Lose Weight," *The Daily Mail Online*, January 1, 2013, http://www.dailymail.co.uk/health/article-2255442/ The-REAL-reason-eat-New-theory-revolutionise-way-lose-weight.html Accessed November 25, 2014.

44 Cummings, David E., MD, et al, "Plasma Ghrelin Levels After Diet-Induced Weight Loss or Gastric Bypass Surgery," *The New England Journal of Medicine,* May 23, 2002, 346:1623-1630. http://www.nejm.org/doi/ full/10.1056/NEJMoa012908

Dr Mark Hyman, author of *The Blood Sugar Solution*, teaches the epigenetic effects of our food consumption. Specifically, he states: "The right food turns on the right genes, and creates biological signals that create health, while the wrong foods turn on genes that cause disease and create biological chaos."[45]

As other health researchers put it, food is processed by our bodies as information that speaks to our genes. David Ludwig, a leading obesity researcher at Harvard Medical School, says, "Molecular pathways involved in hormone action (like insulin resistance) have been the target of a multi-billion-dollar pharmaceutical research effort. However, many of these pathways may normally be under dietary regulation." In other words, what we eat either promotes metabolic health, or its opposite.

Don't feel like you lack willpower or that you are a failure in your inability to keep your weight under control. It's not your fault any more than it would be if you suffered from any other disorder like high blood pressure or cancer or rheumatoid arthritis. This is a medical disorder and, happily, it can be addressed successfully.

Armed with the knowledge that an obstructed airway, sleep apnea, and poor sleep may be at the core of your weight problems, you can take control of the situation. That deeply entrenched vicious cycle can be broken and you will see that it has nothing to do with willpower.

» **Action: See a dentist and have your airway checked.** Be fitted for an oral appliance that moves your jaw forward and keeps the tongue aligned to open the airway during sleep.

» **Action: Get a sleep study, in-home or at a sleep study center.**

» **Action: Consider a CPAP machine.** CPAP machines have been shown to ameliorate many of the problems associated with sleep apnea.

---

45 Hyman, Mark, MD, "Eating the Cure – Mark Hyman, MD in 24/7 Magazine With Bonus Podcast," August 3, 2012, http://drhyman.com/blog/2012/08/03/eating-the-cure-mark-hyman-md-in-24seven-magazine-with-bonus-podcast/#close Accessed November 25, 2014.

» **Action: Avoid having teeth pulled, as this shrinks the jaw.**

» **Action: Follow a regular program of good sleep hygiene (see Chapter 13).**

7

CHAPTER

Women & Sleep-Disordered Breathing

One of the most incredible women I have ever met is Nancy, a 74-year-old from Virginia. She came into the office complaining about back pain, headaches, neck pain, sinusitis and fatigue. You can see by her photo that she was worn out, looking haggard with small, bloodshot eyes and pale skin.

LATERAL
BEFORE AND AFTER

Pre-Treatment
2-2009

Progress
1-2013

Like most of my patients with multiple chronic symptoms, Nancy was suffering from a lack of oxygen and deep restorative sleep. Her Cone Beam CT scan demonstrated a narrowed airway, bone on bone temporomandibular joints, and a small, retruded jaw. Within months of opening her airway with Airway Centric® oral appliances Nancy was feeling rejuvenated with little to no pain. No back pain, no neck pain and no headaches. Her airway size had grown more than six times. Her eyes were open and brighter and her skin glowed with fewer wrinkles. She had a joie de vivre.

At age 80, Nancy continues to have an upbeat spirit with a terrific sense of humor and over 60 years of marriage to a wonderful man. Her facial morphs continue to bring hope to 74-year-old women who now believe in looking and feeling 10 to 15 years younger with a recognition of airway sleep disorders and increased oxygen and deeper sleep.

Detecting Sleep-Disordered Breathing in Women

If you are like many women, you may not even realize that you have a form of sleep-disordered breathing, especially if you don't snore, or if you don't have a bed partner to tell you whether or not you snore. So many of us have stress- or pain-related issues with sleeping—especially as we age—that we often consider our sleep problems to be "normal."

Kelly Brown, MD, Professor of Clinical Neurology at Vanderbilt Sleep Center warns that sleep-disordered breathing in women often goes undiagnosed, in part because of the expectation that sleep apnea "is a disease of middle-aged men."[1] While the prevalence of sleep apnea in men has been measured as high as 30%, the prevalence in women has been measured at 15%.[2] One study suggests, however, that 93% of women with "signs and symptoms of moderate to severe sleep-disordered breathing remain undiagnosed."[3]

---

1 Pashricha, Trisha, "Undiagnosed Sleep Apnea among Women on Rise," *Vanderbilt University Medical Center Reporter*, Posted on Thursday, Mar. 27, 2014 – 8:26 AM. http://news.vanderbilt.edu/2014/03/undiagnosed-sleep-apnea-among-women-on-rise/

2 Ibid.

3 Prasad, Bharati, Janet B. Croft, and Yong Liu, "Sleep-Disordered Breathing," in *Breathing in America: Diseases, Progress, and Hope*, Dean E. Schraufnagel, MD, editor, 2010, American Thoracic Society, p. 239. http://www.thoracic.org/education/breathing-in-america/resources/chapter-23-sleep-disordered-breathing.pdf

Dr Brown notes that women often feel embarrassed to admit that they snore. She further explains that one reason sleep-apnea is under-diagnosed in women is that their symptoms—which include snoring, snorting or nighttime "choking"—can differ from men's. In contrast, women more often report fatigue, morning headaches and depression.[4]

While men often report excessive daytime sleepiness, women more typically report insomnia. Dr Brown explains that women may have an apneic event without realizing what awakened them. Taking a sleeping pill to go back to sleep, she adds, may actually exacerbate the sleep apnea.

Upper airway resistance syndrome (UARS) is a form of sleep-disordered breathing more common in women. Its symptoms can be virtually identical with functional somatic disorders like fibromyalgia and chronic fatigue, as well as anxiety disorders including depression.

According to Dr Brown, sleep apnea may be an underlying cause for refractory migraines, difficult-to-treat hypertension, atrial fibrillation, mood issues or other cognitive concerns.[5] If you experience any of these issues, consider getting a sleep study.

Dr Avram Gold, Director of the Sleep Disorders Center of the State University of New York at Stony Brook, introduced the notion that sleep-disordered breathing often underlies functional somatic syndromes, which are more often experienced by women.

Dr Gold also suggests that SDBs underlie many anxiety disorders.[6] Specifically, he theorizes that sleep-disordered breathing creates a stress response which activates the HPA axis (hypothalamic-pituitary-adrenal axis), which in turn creates an unhealthy imbalance of hormones and a negative effect on the autonomic nervous system.[7]

---

4 Pashricha, Trisha.

5 Ibid.

6 Gold, Avram, MD, "Functional Somatic Syndromes, Anxiety Disorders and the Upper Airway: A Matter of Paradigms," *Sleep Medicine Reviews*, Volume 15, Issue 6, pages 389-401, December 2011.

7 Ibid.

Since women more often than men experience chronic fatigue, and since there may be a link between such conditions and SDBs, we invite you to consider Dr Gold's lists of syndromes, which he theorizes may be linked to SDBs:

- Chronic fatigue
- Fibromyalgia
- Restless legs syndrome
- Irritable bowel syndrome
- Migraine/tension headache syndrome
- Temporomandibular joint syndrome
- Mitral valve prolapse syndrome
- War-related illness (Gulf War syndrome)
- Multiple chemical sensitivity (sick house syndrome)
- Joint hypermobility syndrome[8]

Dr Gold also lists the following anxiety disorders, which often include SDBs, as an underlying factor:

- Panic disorder
- Generalized anxiety disorder
- Social phobia
- Post-traumatic stress disorder
- Obsessive-compulsive disorder[9]

If you have any of the above conditions, we recommend that you get tested for sleep-disordered breathing, because the reduced oxygen while sleeping, along with the effects of sleep fragmentation, may be aggravating your overall condition.

Many women tend to just live with their suffering, taking care of everyone else, but rarely getting around caring for themselves. If you are in pain; feel fatigued; or if you experience insomnia, stress, depression, or anxiety, you may have sleep-disordered breathing, and you deserve to get relief. Even if you do not snore, you may be mouth breathing or have upper airway resistance syndrome, which is harder to detect, but may be causing many of your symptoms.

---

8 Ibid.
9 Ibid.

Upper Airway Resistance Syndrome

One researcher found that 56% of those who suffer from upper airway resistance syndrome are women, and nearly one-third are of East Asian origin. Common characteristics of women with upper airway resistance syndrome include: young to middle-aged, thin to normal weight, blacking out/fainting/dizziness upon standing, wisdom teeth removed at a young age, an overbite (overjet – top teeth farther out than bottom teeth), anxiety, low blood pressure and cold extremities.[10] If you have any of these symptoms, you may have upper airway resistance syndrome.

One study found that obese women with OSA had higher incidences of pre-eclampsia and diabetes, and were about twice as likely to need a Caesarean section. Babies born to pregnant women with OSA are more often born with low birth weight, lower Apgar scores, and more likely to need neonatal intensive care.

Upper airway resistance syndrome (UARS) is a subtle, partial blockage of the airway due to relaxation and partial collapse of the tissues in the throat. Many sleep centers do not even test for this SDB, but it is a very real condition, marked by one very notable characteristic: people with UARS tend to exhibit what is called alpha-delta sleep.[11]

Alpha-delta sleep can occur when a person's brain is triggered by respiratory effort-related arousals (RERAs), when sensitive receptors in the throat perceive a negative pressure in the airway (as occurs in UARS), so that the brain goes from the deep slow-wave delta sleep into a light alpha stage of sleep, or into actual wakefulness.

Christian Guilleminault, M.D., a research physician at Stanford and an award-winning expert in the field of sleep medicine, notes a distinct difference between people with UARS and people who suffer from obstructive sleep apnea, or OSA. Guilleminault explains that people with UARS experience increased respiratory effort without the type of airway collapse associated with OSA. People who suffer

---

10 Guilleminault, Christian and Susmita Chowdhuri, "Upper Airway Resistance Syndrome Is a Distinct Syndrome," *American Journal of Respiratory and Critical Care Medicine*, Volume 161, No. 5, 1412-1413.

11 Ibid.

from UARS also do not experience the same degree of oxygen de-saturation. Instead, they tend to arouse easily from the respiratory effort, creating the alpha-delta sleep. UARS patients typically report insomnia, sleep fragmentation, and fatigue.[12] Guilleminault and his colleagues state: "In UARS, the arousal threshold is lower."

This is apparently due to the receptors in the throats of UARS patients being far more sensitive than the receptors in the throats of patients with obstructive sleep apnea. This leads to different sleep patterns: more delta sleep with alpha intrusions in UARS, and less delta with more stages 1 and 2 in OSA. In UARS and OSA, the autonomic nervous system reacts very differently; in OSA, it is overly activated and leads to hypertension, while in UARS it is under-activated and hypotension (low blood pressure) is common.[13]

In other words, if you snore mildly, or even if you do not snore, and if you experience insomnia, sometimes black-out or feel faint when standing, have normal to low blood pressure, wake easily during the night, and feel fatigued when you wake up, you may have UARS.

Dr Avram Gold says that the symptoms of UARS and the symptoms of functional somatic syndrome disorders such as fibro-myalgia are very similar.[14] Since both UARS and functional somatic disorders occur more often in women, more research into the possible links could be helpful for identifying effective treatments.

We know, for instance, that SDBs in general can lead to increased inflammation. Researchers at the Washington University School of Medicine found that there are links between inflamma-tion and restless leg syndrome. They also note that inflammation is associated with chronic fatigue, fibromyalgia, and irritable bowel syndrome.[15] Since all of these functional somatic disorders involve inflammation, and since UARS and other forms of SDBs create a

---

12 Ibid.

13 Ibid.

14 Gold, Avram, et al, "The Symptoms and Signs of Upper Airway Resistance Syndrome," *Chest Journal*, January 2003, 123:87-95. http://www.chestjournal.org

15 Weinstock, Leonard B., et al, "Restless legs syndrome – Theoret-ical roles of inflammatory and immune mechanisms," *Sleep Medicine Reviews*, XXX (2011), 1-14. http://www.rlcure.com/rls_study.pdf

stress response in the body that can include inflammation, further research is needed to look into possible links, especially research that focuses on identifying UARS in women, along with functional somatic disorders and anxiety disorders.

Pregnancy and Sleep-Disordered Breathing

Pregnancy increases the likelihood of a woman developing sleep-disordered breathing. As one researcher states, "snoring, the most common symptom of sleep-disordered breathing, is markedly increased during pregnancy."[16]

Excessive weight gain during pregnancy, or alternatively the combination of weight gain and obesity during pregnancy, contributes to a higher risk of sleep apnea. During later stages of pregnancy, the upward pressure on the diaphragm can contribute to SDBs. Hormonal changes, particularly an increase in estrogen, can contribute to swelling and congestion in the upper airway, which in turn increase the likelihood of snoring and other SDBs.[17]

As we stated earlier, obstructive sleep apnea and other SDBs have been linked to elevated blood pressure, diabetes, and metabolic syndrome. With pregnancy, these risks create even greater concern, for both the mom and the baby. In fact, research has shown that women who are pregnant and who have SDBs have a greater risk of gestational hypertension and preeclampsia.

One study reviewed the 2003 national survey of Health Care Cost and Utilization, which included data on nearly 4 million pregnant women. This study found that pregnant women with sleep apnea were four times more likely to develop pregnancy-induced hypertension, and twice as likely to develop gestational diabetes, than pregnant women without OSA.[18]

The risks of complications for both mother and baby are higher when a woman is both obese and pregnant. Dr Judette Law, lead

---

16 Venkata, Chakradhar, MD, and Saiprakash B. Venkateshiah, MD, "Sleep-Disordered Breathing During Pregnancy," *Journal of the American Board of Family Medicine,* March-April 2009, Vol. 22, No. 2, 158-168. http://jabfm.org/content/22/2/158.full

17 Ibid.

18 Ibid.

author, and a team of researchers at Case Western Reserve studied obese pregnant women with sleep apnea, as well as obese pregnant women without sleep apnea. They found not only higher incidences of preeclampsia and diabetes, but also obese women with OSA were about twice as likely to need a Caesarean section.[19]

The complications of maternal sleep apnea for the baby are also very high risk. The scientists at Case Western Reserve found that the babies of obese pregnant women with sleep apnea were almost three times more likely to need neonatal intensive care than the babies of obese pregnant women without sleep apnea.[20]

The hypoxemia that can result from OSA can lead to slower growth of the fetus. One study even found that 3 out of 4 mothers with OSA delivered babies who had lower birth weights as well as lower Apgar scores (a test of developmental abilities of newborns) than babies of mothers without OSA.[21]

Clearly more research is needed in this area as to how OSA affects the fetus during pregnancy, although a small study did find that the baby's heart rate slowed significantly during the mother's apneic episodes.[22]

Unfortunately, research shows that very low birth weight increases the risk of sleep-disordered breathing when that infant becomes a young adult. So, if a pregnant woman has untreated sleep-disordered breathing, and gives birth to a low-birth-weight baby, that baby is more likely to develop SDBs as a young adult.[23]

---

19 Louis, Judette, MD, MPH, et al, "Perinatal Outcomes Associated with Obstructive Sleep Apnea in Obese Pregnant Women," *Obstetrics & Gynecology,* November 2012, Volume 120, Issue 5, pp. 1085-1092. http://journals.lww.com/greenjournal/Fulltext/2012/11000/Perinatal_Outcomes_Associated_With_Obstructive.15.aspx. Also discussed here: http://www.dailymail.co.uk/health/article-2206267/Sleep-apnoea-pregnancy-harm-health-mother-baby.html#ixzz2sepcKtUy

20 Ibid.

21 Ibid.

22 http://www.sharecare.com/health/health-pregnancy/how-sleep-apnea-affect-baby

23 Paavonen, EJ, et al, "Very low birth weight increases risk for sleep-disordered breathing in young adults: The Helsinki Study of Very

Finally, that same research found that if a woman smokes during pregnancy, her child's risk of developing sleep-disordered breathing as a young adult actually doubles.[24] With pregnancy, the cycle of sleep-disordered breathing, if untreated, can continue from generation to generation.

Pregnancy and Preventing SDBs

If you are thinking about becoming pregnant, and if you think you might have some form of sleep-disordered breathing, we recommend that you get a sleep study at a center that tests for UARS. If you have some form of SDB, we recommend that you get it treated.

Before becoming pregnant, we recommend that you seek to attain or maintain a healthy weight, address any issues that may contribute to nasal congestion, and have an Airway Centric® dentist evaluate your teeth and jaw for any potential airway issues.

During pregnancy, be sure to keep your weight gain within healthy limits, and avoid alcohol and other drugs that might decrease your sleep quality and directly increase health risks for your baby. If you suspect that you have developed OSA during pregnancy, get a sleep study and treat even mild OSA with a CPAP machine to avoid oxygen deprivation in your baby.

Oral appliances can be helpful for treating SDBs during pregnancy, but because they require adjustments over a period of time, the ideal time to be fitted for an oral appliance is before pregnancy.

Menopause and SDBs

One set of researchers actually refer to menopause as a risk factor for SDBs in women.[25] Although research needs to be developed to study the link between menopause and the development of SDBs, the suggestion is that decreasing estrogen levels during menopause often cause women to develop sleep apnea.

Low Birth Weight Adults," Pediatrics, October 2007, 120 (4); 778-84. http://www.ncbi.nlm.nih.gov/pubmed/17908765

24 Ibid.

25 Prasad, Bharati, et al.

Both estrogen and progesterone "maintain the airway and keep it from collapsing."[26]

One study found that perimenopausal women are eight times more likely to develop sleep apnea than either premenopausal or postmenopausal women. Another study found that postmenopausal women who do not receive hormone replacement therapy are five times more likely to develop sleep apnea.[27]

Weight gain is also often associated with menopause, and as we have stated before, weight gain alone can contribute to the development of SDBs.

If you are perimenopausal, menopausal, or postmenopausal, experiencing weight gain, foggy thinking, elevated blood pressure, hot flashes at night, night sweats, or morning migraines, the root of your problems may be sleep-disordered breathing. We recommend that you get a sleep study, treat your sleep apnea or other SDB accordingly, and discuss the possibility of hormone replacement therapy, particularly natural HRT, with your physician.

Breast Cancer and Sleep-Disordered Breathing

While research on this subject is still needed, we know that sleep disruption also adversely affects the immune system, potentially opening the door to cancer.[28] Studies have shown that women who sleep less than six hours per night are more likely to develop breast cancer than women who sleep longer.[29] The brainwave patterns and body chemistry changes due to shorter sleep duration are very similar to the changes that occur with sleep-disordered breathing.

---

26 http://sleepdisorders.about.com/od/causesofsleepdisorder1/fl/Menopause-and-the-Risk-of-Sleep-Apnea-in-Women.htm

27 http://www.34-menopause-symptoms.com/sleep-disorders/articles/understanding-sleep-apnea.htm

28 See, for instance, Gozal, David, "Fragmented Sleep Accelerates Cancer Growth," University of Chicago Medical Center, as reported on *Science Daily.* http://www.sciencedaily.com/releases/2014/01/140127100947.htm

29 See Brody, Jane, above, endnote 109.

Now, top sleep doctors are suggesting there is a link between sleep-disordered breathing and breast cancer. Dr Kelly Brown of Vanderbilt University Medical Center notes that both disrupted sleep and obesity, which are common in sleep apnea patients, are risk factors for breast cancer.[30] One study shows that women with breast cancer who experience fragmented sleep have higher mortality rates than women with breast cancer who sleep well.[31]

Dr Steven Park, author of *Sleep, Interrupted*, makes the case for the physiological link between sleep-disordered breathing and breast cancer. Dr Park has examined many patients with breast cancer and found several commonalities among them, most notably very small airways. Dr Park's theory about the connection between SDBs and breast cancer involves several physiological mechanisms. One is the physiological stress caused by SDBs, linking to inhibited blood flow to extremities such as hands and feet, as well as breast tissues, thus reducing the oxygen present in the tissues.[32]

Further research into the possible connection between breast cancer and sleep-disordered breathing is much needed. In the meantime, if you have breast cancer, we recommend that you have a sleep study and treat any SDBs in order to enhance your body's immune system and increase your body's ability to heal and to prevent recurrence.

---

30 Pashricha, Trisha.

31 Palesh, Oxana, et al, "Sleep Disruption Predicts Survival of Women with Advanced Breast Cancer," *Sleep* 2014, 37(5):837-842. http://www.journalsleep.org/ViewAbstract.aspx?pid=29448

32 http://doctorstevenpark.com/sleep-apnea-and-breast-cancer-is-there-a-connection and also: http://doctorstevenpark.com/breast-cancer-and-the-sleep-apnea%E2%80%93alcohol-link

8

C H A P T E R

Mental Health and Blocked Airways

Which Came First: Mental Health Challenges or Poor Sleep?

We all struggle with anxiety during difficult times in our lives—a loved one becomes ill, we get laid off from a job, finances spin out of control, or a marriage falls apart. Certainly these stressors cause anxiety—that fight-or-flight response that makes us irritable, edgy and impatient—but generally these are temporary set-backs and the anxiety goes away when the situation improves.

If you suffer from ongoing anxiety or depression, you are far from alone. Anxiety disorders represent the most common form of mental challenge in the United States, affecting 40 million adults or 18% or the population aged 18 and older.[1] Depression affects 7-9% of the population, or at least 16 million adults.[2] Anxiety and

1 According to the Anxiety and Depression Association of America website: http://www.adaa.org/about-adaa/press-room/facts-statistics

2 The National Institutes of Mental Health reports 6.9% in 2012 (http://www.nimh.nih.gov/statistics/1mdd_adult.shtml), while the Centers for Disease Control reports 9.1% in 2006 and 2008 (http://www.cdc.gov/features/dsdepression/)

depression are the most common chronic illnesses in people who have sleep-disordered breathing.

Researchers commonly find that sleep-disordered breathing is associated with a variety of mental challenges: ADHD in children and adults, anxiety, depression, irritability, memory deficits, inability to concentrate, and decreased alertness.[3] Moreover, people who are deeply depressed are almost six times more likely to report having severe sleep apnea than are healthy people.[4]

Even worse, according to Dr Vatsal G. Thakkar, clinical assistant professor of psychiatry at the NYU School of Medicine, adults with sleep deficits or disrupted sleep are often misdiagnosed as having ADHD, when in reality, their only problem is needing a good night's sleep.[5]

Imagine repeatedly being suffocated at night while you're trying to sleep. Terrifying, isn't it? That's what people with sleep apnea deal with all night, every night, even though they may not be aware of it. Naturally, this leads to a physiological stress response, aka: anxiety.

Sleep interruption leads to fragmented sleep architecture, meaning the cycle of progressively deeper sleep stages is broken. Snoring causes the sleeper to reset to stage 1, the lightest sleep stage. The deepest REM sleep might never be reached if airways are blocked and there is snoring. This gets the defense mechanisms locked and loaded, ready for fight or flight. But the only "enemy" is the poor, defenseless obstructed airway.

People with OSA therefore wake up feeling lethargic, yet anxious. All day long they are nervous and startle easily. Panic attacks set in over seemingly small issues. It's hard to think clearly. Anxiety becomes chronic and difficult to manage.

---

3 Flemons, W. Ward, MD, and Willis Tsai, MD, "Quality of Life Consequences of Sleep-Disordered Breathing," *Journal of Allergy and Clinical Immunology,* Vol. 99, Issue 2, February 1997, 5750-5756.

4 Cheng, P., et al, "Sleep-Disordered Breathing in Major Depressive Disorder," *Journal of Sleep Research*, August 2013, 22 (4), 459-62. http://www.ncbi.nlm.nih.gov/pubmed/23350718

5 Thakkar, Vatsal, G., MD, "Diagnosing the Wrong Deficit," *The New York Times,* April 27, 2013. http://www.nytimes.com/2013/04/28/opinion/sunday/diagnosing-the-wrong-deficit.html?_r=0

Anxiety and depression are often accompanied by insomnia—when it is difficult to fall and stay asleep. When the nervous system is in high gear, it is hard to shut off. Because SDBs start this chronic pattern of anxiety and depression, we suggest that SDBs often precede the development of insomnia. Unlike other chronic diseases, anxiety and depression are not caused by inflammation, but they are strongly connected to SDB and OSA. The fear of suffocating is primal and universal, and the anxiety it causes lasts throughout the day.

Scientific evidence comes from University of Iowa researchers who studied a woman whose amygdala, the brain's fear center, was damaged. She experienced no anxiety, even when threatened by snakes, spiders, robbers, haunted houses and horror films. However, when scientists had her inhale a harmless amount of carbon dioxide she experienced anxiety for the first time. They found the same results with two other women whose amygdalas were damaged.[6]

> **People with SDBs** have brains that may be experiencing a state of panic off-and-on all night long, so they wake up lethargic but anxious. That anxiety becomes chronic and difficult to manage.

Here's the connection to sleep apnea: during apneas and hypopneas, the brain's oxygen level decreases, and the level of carbon dioxide in the blood often increases. While people are sleeping, this same internal fear system gets triggered as was triggered in these women because the brain panics when it does not get enough oxygen.

If you're hoping for good news, here it is: researchers have found that treating patients with mental challenges for their sleep-disordered breathing can actually bring them relief. For instance, a group of researchers found that treating patients who have sleep apnea with a CPAP machine led to improvement of their mood disorders from OSA, as well as their ability to think, to focus, and to perform

---

6 Gorman, James, "Study Discovers Internal Trigger for Panic Attack in the Previously Fearless," February 3, 2013, *The New York Times.* http://www.nytimes.com/2013/02/04/health/study-discovers-internal-trigger-for-the-previously-fearless.html?_r=0

mental tasks.[7] We see these results with our patients as well, when we fit them with a custom dental appliance to help keep their airways open.

Dr Thakkar writes that the FDA recently approved giving patients with ADHD the drug clonidine, although many psychiatrists don't realize that the very reason it works is that clonidine induces delta sleep (deep restorative sleep).[8] Similarly, addressing sleep-disordered breathing can bring relief to people with ADHD, anxiety, and depression, because keeping the airway open at night allows them to maintain adequate periods of deep delta wave sleep as well as REM sleep.

Researchers at Harvard have noted that many people with psychiatric disorders have sleep issues. In the July 2009 issue of the *Harvard Mental Health Letter*, they state: "Chronic sleep problems affect 50-80% of patients in a typical psychiatric practice, compared with 10-18% of adults in the general U.S. population. Sleep problems are particularly common in patients with anxiety, depression, bipolar disorder, and attention deficit hyperactivity disorder (ADHD)." They raise the issue that for both children and adults, sleep disorders, including sleep apnea, "may actually contribute to psychiatric disorders."[9]

Their estimates of the prevalence of sleep issues among people with mental disorders included 70 potential sleep problems, the most common of which are: insomnia, sleep apnea, movement disorders such as restless legs syndrome, and narcolepsy. Yet, as mentioned earlier, we know that sleep-disordered breathing can lead to insomnia, so SDB may even be an unknown yet underlying factor in many cases of insomnia as well.

When considering the prevalence of sleep-disordered breathing among people with health issues of any sort, including mental health issues, most researchers only look for the presence of

---

7 Flemons, et al.

8 Thakkar, Vatsal.

9 "Sleep and Mental Health," *Harvard Mental Health Letter,* July 2009. Available online at:

http://www.health.harvard.edu/newsletters/Harvard_Mental_Health_Letter/2009/July/Sleep-and-mental-health sleep apnea. Unfortunately, there persists a lack of awareness that sleep-disordered breathing also includes mouth breathing, simple snoring, hypopneas, and upper airway resistance syndrome. There is a serious need for further research on the connection between all forms of SDBs and mental health.

Post-Traumatic Stress Disorder and Sleep-Disordered Breathing

A study of veterans referred for sleep studies proves the point that awareness of all the forms of SDBs could bring about different research outcomes. While they did find a connection between OSA—both mild and moderate to severe, with anxiety—they primarily found a link between insomnia and PTSD. However, they included snorers in their control group, and most of the patients with insomnia were women, suggesting that they probably did not test for UARS. This is noteworthy since this group also reported high levels of pain syndromes. The fact that they found a link between insomnia and PTSD is, nonetheless, significant.[10]

Other researchers have found a connection between sleep apnea and PTSD. As a matter of fact, a 2005 study of over four million veterans found a link between sleep apnea and several mental disorders: PTSD, anxiety, depression, psychosis, and bi-polar disorder. The researchers found a "significantly greater prevalence" of each of these disorders among veterans with OSA than among veterans without sleep apnea. Given the very large sample size, these are significant findings.[11]

Research such as this has led the Department of Veterans Affairs to treat OSA as a consequence of PTSD in some cases,[12]

---

10 Mysliwiec, Vincent, MD, et al, "Sleep Disorders and Associated Medical Comorbidities in Active Duty Personnel," *Sleep*, 2013, Volume 36, Issue 2, 167-174. http://www.journalsleep.org/ViewAbstract.aspx?pid=28780

11 Sharafkhaneh, Amir, MD, et al, "Association of Psychiatric Disorders and Sleep Apnea in a Large Cohort," *Sleep*, Vol. 28, No. 11, 2005, 1405-1411. http://www.journalsleep.org/Articles/281111.pdf

12 http://www.va.gov/vetapp01/files01/0102100.txt

but not in others,[13] and indeed, there may be a bi-directional re-lationship. Some researchers have raised the issue that perhaps sleep apnea precedes and contributes to the development of PTSD.

Dr Robert S. Rosenberg, a sleep medicine specialist, asks the question: "If the sleep apnea were coincidental or secondary, why is it that treating the sleep disorder results in significant improvement in the anxiety disorder?" Instead, Dr Rosenberg suggests that sleep apnea pre-exists the anxiety disorders, and therefore contributes to their development.

We strongly recommend that you obtain a sleep study if you have been diagnosed with PTSD, or if you suspect that you may have PTSD from trauma during war, sexual assault, or other experiences of violence or emotional abuse. Ensuring your brain and body receive a good night's sleep is a vital first step on the path to healing and recovery from any form of trauma.

Dr Rosenberg is addressing both the PTSD found among veterans, as well as the PTSD found among women who have experienced the traumatic violence of sexual assault. His theory rests on the role of the limbic system in the brain, especially the role of the amygdala and the fight-flight-freeze response.[14]

In other words, Dr Rosenberg's theory offers similar insight into the research of Dr Avram Gold. You may recall from the chapter on women and sleep-disordered breathing that Dr Gold suggests that sleep-disordered breathing may be the original stressful condition that leads to exacerbated mental and physiological conditions due to the body's stress response. Importantly, Dr Gold's model of sleep-disordered breathing, stress response, and both anxiety disorders and functional somatic disorders predicts that use of a CPAP machine for relief of these stress-related disorders will not be immediate, but will occur after a few months of use.

Dr Rosenberg concurs: veterans who use CPAP machines often stop using them because they do not see immediate results.

---

13 http://www.va.gov/vetapp10/files3/1025438.txt

14 Rosenberg, Robert S., MD, "The PTSD and Sleep Apnea Connection," http://www.answersforsleep.com/sleep-and-neurological-dis-orders/the-ptsd-and-sleep-apnea-connection/

However, Dr Rosenberg contends that, with continued use of a CPAP machine, over time, veterans can see improvement in their symptoms, even of PTSD and their daytime symptoms.[15]

If you have been diagnosed with PTSD, or if you suspect that you may have PTSD from war trauma, sexual assault, or other violence or emotional abuse, then request a sleep-study. If you have PTSD and any form of sleep-disordered breathing, we recommend that you get fitted with a CPAP machine and/or a dental appliance designed to open your airway at night. Ensuring your brain and body receive a good night's sleep is a vital first step on the path to healing and recovery from any form of trauma.

Alzheimer's Disease and Sleep-Disordered Breathing

Researchers at the New York University School of Medicine found an association between sleep-disordered breathing and biological brain changes that increase risk of Alzheimer's in thin senior adults. Although the study was not longitudinal and therefore cannot speak to the development of Alzheimer's, in thin seniors, the presence of disruptive breathing during sleep was found to be associated with both brain damage and decreased use of glucose by the brain.[16]

There may in fact be a physiological link between sleep apnea and Alzheimer's disease. Researchers at Stanford University's Center for Human Sleep Research have found that people with a certain genetic marker called APOE4 are twice as likely to suffer from sleep apnea as people who do not have this genetic marker. APOE4 also predisposes people to the development of Alzheimer's. However, this does not mean that if you have sleep apnea, you will necessarily develop Alzheimer's; it simply means there is an increased risk among those who have sleep apnea and those who have the genetic marker APOE4.[17]

15 Ibid.

16 Dotinga, Randy, HealthDay Reporter, "Sleep Apnea in Seniors Tied to Alzheimer's in Study," *US News & World Report Health*, May 19, 2013, online. http://health.usnews.com/health-news/news/articles/2013/05/19/sleep-apnea-in-seniors-tied-to-alzheimers-in-study

17 Eisner, Robin, "Study: Snoring, Alzheimer's Link?" abcnews.com June 13, 2014 http://abcnews.go.com/Health/story?id=117398

If you are nonetheless wondering if there is any hope of preventing Alzheimer's in yourself or someone you love, there is hope. Researchers have recently discovered what they call a "glymphatic system," which flushes toxins out of the brain while we sleep.[18]

As explained by neuroscientists at the University of Rochester Medical Center, the neurons in our brains shrink by 60% while we sleep, thus allowing cerebrospinal fluid to flush the toxins out of our brains. This function is similar to the lymphatic system, which flushes toxins out of the body; however, in the brain, the flushing happens between the nerve cells, and among the glial cells, so they dubbed it the "glymphatic system."

Lead researcher Dr Maiken Nedergaard explains that this process can only happen while we sleep, not while we are awake. "You can think of it like having a house party. You can either entertain the guests or clean up the house, but you can't really do both at the same time."[19]

We can extrapolate from this that the nightly disruptions from SDBs, including respiratory-effort related arousals, oxygen deprivations, hypoxemia, sleep fragmentation such that deep sleep is disrupted, full awakenings, alpha-delta sleep, and so on, would interfere with this nightly pattern of shrinking neurons and flushing the brain of toxins.

Autism and Sleep-Disordered Breathing

Autism has been increasing at alarming rates over the last 20 years or more. According to the Centers for Disease Control, one in 68 children in the US now has an autism spectrum disorder. This represents a 30% increase from just two years earlier.[20] In the 1970s

---

18 Duff, Kat, "While We Sleep, Neurotoxins Are Flushed Away," December 4, 2013, The Secret Life of Sleep. http://www.thesecret-lifeofsleep.com/2013/12/

19 Ibid.

20 Falco, Miriam, "Autism Rates Now 1 in 68 US Children: CDC," CNN. com, March 28, 2014. http://www.cnn.com/2014/03/27/health/cdc-autism/

and 1980s, 1 in 2,000 children was labeled autistic.[21] Granted, much of the increase may represent an increase in diagnosis, but clearly this is an astounding increase. Scientists have not yet agreed on what causes autism.[22]

If you have a child with autism, you know that this one diagnosis often comes with a whole variety of issues that busy parents somehow need to address. Sleep problems are only one of the many issues that affect parents of children with autism spectrum disorders, with the child's sleep issues often impacting the parents' ability to get a good night's sleep as well.

Dr Gail Williams, M.D., Associate Professor of Pediatrics and Clinical Co-Director of the University of Louisville Autism Center, informs us that 50-80% of children with autism spectrum disorder experience sleep problems, as compared to 9-50% of normally-developing children experiencing sleep problems.[23]

Operating primarily out of the paradigm that autism contributes to these sleep problems, rather than a paradigm that sees a potential bi-directional relationship between the two, Dr Williams recommends treating the array of problems that typically arise, in part, because of SDBs such as anxiety, depression, GERD, and insomnia. Dr Williams does helpfully recommend that sleep-disordered breathing be treated, including recommending removal of children's tonsils and adenoids to prevent OSA.

As expressed in earlier chapters, we know there is research suggesting that SDBs may contribute to all the above conditions, so parents who may be struggling to deal with their child's autistic issues may wish to focus on addressing any potential sleep-disordered breathing sooner rather than later in order to improve as many symptoms as possible. Also, as mentioned earlier, insomnia

---

21 Doheny, Kathleen, "Autism Cases on the Rise; Reason for Increase a Mystery," WebMD, 2014. http://www.webmd.com/brain/autism/searching-for-answers/autism-rise

22 Ibid.

23 Williams, Gail, "Sleep Problems in Children with Autism," University of Kentucky Autism Center, Fall 2011. http://louisville.edu/education/kyautismtraining/about/newsletters/sleep-problems-in-children-with-autism

may arise from sleep-disordered breathing, so treating any SDBs a child may have may help prevent issues with insomnia as well.

A comprehensive article on possible causes of autism written by a former pharmaceutical researcher, Helen Ratajczak, was published in the *Journal of Immunotoxicology* in 2011. In this article, Dr Ratajczak writes: "Autism could result from more than one cause, with different manifestations in different individuals that share common symptoms. Documented causes of autism include genetic mutations and/or deletions, viral infections, and encephalitis following vaccination. Therefore, autism is the result of genetic defects and/or inflammation of the brain. The inflammation could be caused by a defective placenta, immature blood-brain barrier, the immune response of the mother to infection while pregnant, a premature birth, encephalitis in the child after birth, or a toxic environment."[24]

> **Inflammation of the brain** is often involved in the development of autism, so preventing and treating SDBs, which contribute to inflammation, could be vitally important for improving mental and physical health outcomes for individuals with autism spectrum disorders.

What is relevant to our purposes here in exploring the role of the airway is that inflammation of the brain is often involved in the development of autism. Sleep-disordered breathing often interferes with the body's ability to reduce inflammation, so preventing and treating SDBs in children and adults with autism could be extremely vital to improving their mental and physical health outcomes.

Dr Steven Park reports on a theory of a possible cause of autism that is potentially directly related to airway-centered disorders and SDBs. In November, 2009, Dr Park reports on the theory of

---

24 Ratajczak, HV, "Theoretical Aspects of Autism: Causes – A Review," *Journal of Immunotoxicology,* Jan-Mar 2011; 8 (1): 68-79. http://www.ncbi. nlm.nih.gov/pubmed/21299355 For a very informative interview with Dr Ratajczak, providing further clarity of the issues, including her research techniques, personal motivation for studying autism, and recommendations for further research, please go here: http://www.ageofautism. com/2011/05/autisms-causes-and-biomarkers-an-interview-with-helen-ratajczak-phd.html

Thomas McCabe, who suggests that infants lying on their backs are more susceptible to sleep-disordered breathing, and thus to a lack of healthy brain development. McCabe ties the "back to sleep" campaign, originating in 1992, with the high incidence of autism. While rates of SIDS deaths did decline significantly due to this trend in having infants sleep on their backs, the rate of autism increased at the same time.[25]

More research is clearly needed to assess whether or not infants sleeping on their backs experience more sleep-disordered breathing. Certainly, in adults, sleeping on one's back contributes to worsening any existing sleep-disordered breathing. If your child has been diagnosed with autism, you may want to encourage him or her to become a side-sleeper rather than a back-sleeper.

Down Syndrome and Sleep-Disordered Breathing

Individuals with Down syndrome have higher than average rates of sleep problems. The New York-based National Down Syndrome Society claims that 50-100% of individuals with Down syndrome have obstructive sleep apnea, and almost 60% of children with Down syndrome develop sleep problems by the age of three-and-a-half to four years.[26]

A British study found that children with Down syndrome, when compared with normally-developing children, were much more likely to: mouth-breathe while sleeping, snore, experience episodes of apnea, choking, and gasping. The children with Down syndrome were also far more likely to sleep with their necks extended (one way the brain may compensate to keep the airway open), to wet their beds (can occur with SDBs), and to sleep-walk (this may also be a "side-effect" of SDBs).[27]

25 Park, Steven, MD, November 5, 2009. http://doctorstevenpark.com/intriguing-sleep-apnea-and-autism-connections

26 National Down Syndrome Society, 2012: http://www.ndss.org/Resources/Health-Care/Associated-Conditions/Obstructive-Sleep-Apnea-Down-Syndrome/

27 Stores, R., Stores, G. and Buckley, S. (1996). The pattern of sleep problems in children with Down syndrome and other intellectual disabilities. *Journal of Applied Research in Intellectual Disabilities*, 9(2), 145-158. As reported in an article by Wood, A., and Sacks, B.

A variety of anatomical traits may account for the higher than normal occurrence of SDBs in individuals with Down syndrome: low muscle tone in the face, cheeks, throat, tongue, and jaws; obesity; narrow passages in the nose and throat; poor muscle coordination for breathing and swallowing; narrow jaw/large tongue; and enlarged tonsils and adenoids.[28]

For people with Down syndrome, working with an OMT (orofacial myofunctional therapist) may be necessary to improve muscle tone as well as aid in the coordination of breathing and swallowing properly both night and day. Achieving and maintaining a healthy weight can be beneficial for decreasing the chance of SDBs as well.

If a sleep study is performed and an individual is fitted with a CPAP machine or a dental night guard, we strongly recommend also working with an OMT to improve muscle tone along with proper swallowing and breathing. The combined approach may be essential for improved coordination as well increasing the chance of maintaining open airways.

More research is needed for individuals with Down syndrome and SDBs to find optimal treatment plans so individuals with Down syndrome can maintain compliance and experience a better night's sleep.

"Overcoming sleep problems for children with Down syndrome," Down Syndrome News and Update, 2004; 3 (4); 118-127, available online at: http://www.down-syndrome.org/reviews/320/

28 National Down Syndrome Society, 2012: http://www.ndss.org/ Resources/Health-Care/Associated-Conditions/Obstructive-Sleep-Apnea- -Down-Syndrome/

9

CHAPTER

Chronic Pain, Inflammation, and Your Airway

Nancy, 38 years of age, was referred to us by her father, a dentist. She told us she had been experiencing severe pain and clicking in the left side of her jaw for four years and eating was particularly painful. In further conversation, she told us she had severe lower back pain and migraines.

Upon examination, we found Nancy's jaw and chin were misaligned to the left with a noticeable click in the left temporomandibular joint (the joint between the cranium and the jaw) on the left side. We gave her two appliances, one for daytime use that repositioned her lower jaw and helped realign her chin to the center of her face, and another for nighttime use that maintained this position at night; both were intended to relieve the pain, clicking and popping.

Two weeks later, on her first follow-up visit, Nancy was thrilled that the popping and clicking had completely disappeared, whether she was wearing the appliances or not. At the same visit, Botox was placed in both sides of her jaw-clenching muscles and she reported that her pain disappeared almost immediately and we noticed that her face became even more symmetrical.

In a few more weeks, Nancy's jaw had stabilized in a new centered position where there was no clicking with opening or closing. We also worked with Nancy's father, Ron, who placed laminates on her upper front teeth and onlays on the upper back teeth to give her better contact in the Airway Centric® position so that her airway would stay open day and night.

In addition to giving Nancy a prettier, thinner more symmetrical face we were able to alleviate her chronic pain which had eluded diagnosis. With this simple treatment, Nancy's migraines and back pain completely disappeared. She has now been pain-free for four years.

Pain, Inflammation, and Blocked Airways

Chronic pain affects approximately 100 million Americans; more than the combined number of Americans who have heart disease, cancer, and diabetes.[1] At its root, pain is caused by inflammation. Inflammation can be reduced during deep, restorative sleep, or worsened when SDBs interfere with deep sleep.

Airway obstruction during sleep causes microarousals (MAs), which are 1.5-second to 3-second increases in EEG activity.[2] These MAs in turn increase the heart rate and cause muscle tension. MAs can occur as often as eight to 15 times per hour and each one interrupts the process of reaching those deeper stages of sleep.

These microarousals also increase adrenaline and blood sugar. Then cellular messengers called cytokines signal the body's cells, indicating they are under attack, resulting in inflammation. The inflammatory markers are excited, causing pain.

---

1 Institute of Medicine Report from the Committee on Advancing Pain Research, Care, and Education: *Relieving Pain in America, A Blueprint for Transforming Prevention, Care, Education and Research.* The National Academies Press, 2011. http://books.nap.edu/openbook.php?record_id=13172&page=1

2 Martin, SE, et al, "Microarousals in patients with sleep apnoea/hypopnea syndrome," *Journal of Sleep Research*, 1997, Dec: 6 (4): 276-80. http://www.ncbi.nlm.nih.gov/pubmed/9493529

If you treat the pain but ignore airway function—a rarely considered source of the problem—the pain may simply move to another place, because the inflammatory process has been triggered during disrupted sleep. A compromised airway will likely cause pain somewhere in the body. Living without pain is key to a happy, active life. Without opening an obstructed airway, pain will probably never be completely eliminated.

Less Sleep = More Pain

If you are in pain, it is difficult to sleep. To make matters worse, if you are having trouble sleeping, the pain intensifies. You may feel like you can't win. Researchers have begun to confirm that there is actually a bidirectional relationship between poor sleep quality and pain.

People with fibromyalgia offer a good example: The pain from muscle trigger points (tender points) and the burning sensation and numbness become unbearable, often making it difficult to sleep. It's believed that fibromyalgia amplifies pain sensations by changing how the brain processes pain signals.

A study by Harvey Moldofsky, M.D., of the University of Toronto found fibromyalgia patients' sleep lacked restorative qualities. He showed that stage 4 sleep—the second portion of deep sleep—was fragmented in fibromyalgia patients. Stage 4 sleep is key to stress relief since this is the stage where growth hormone and interleukin—a potent immune modulator—are secreted. Moldofsky found that treating fibromyalgia patients with therapeutic interventions that restore their deep sleep also decreases their pain.[3]

To prove this disruption was the cause of the chronic pain and other symptoms, Moldofsky interrupted the stage 4 sleep of healthy patients. In just a few days, these healthy people experienced pain in the same tender muscle points that fibromyalgia patients experience. Moreover, the healthy patients whose deep sleep was

---

3 Moldofsky, H, MD, "The significance of dysfunctions of the sleeping/ waking brain to the pathogenesis and treatment of fibromyalgia syndrome," *Journal of Rheumatic Diseases Clinics of North America*, May 2009;35(2):275-83. http://www.ncbi.nlm.nih.gov/pubmed/19647142

disrupted showed brain EEG patterns that were similar to the EEGs of patients with fibromyalgia during sleep.[4]

This study and others show that not only does pain cause sleep disruptions, but also disrupted sleep can literally cause pain.

Sleep Disruption, Pain, and Airways

An obstructed airway makes deep sleep difficult to attain and maintain. Moreover, pain medications and sleep aids often disrupt deep sleep and further contribute to sleep-disordered breathing, resulting in slower recovery time from painful injuries and chronic pain.

To reduce pain, first we need to open the airway. We find this time and time again with our patients; opening the airway and reducing sleep-disordered breathing reduces pain. It's as simple as this: pain relief comes from deep sleep, and deep sleep is improved with an open airway.

Headaches

In our experience with patients, waking up with a headache is one of the cardinal signs of sleep apnea as well as of upper airway resistance syndrome. The types of headaches vary: migraine, cluster, hypnic, or just that feeling of a dull achy head.

Morning headaches can stem from many causes, among them sleep apnea, restless leg syndrome, chronic pain and insomnia. Tension, clenched teeth, TMJ, allergies or hormonal imbalance also may contribute to morning headaches, yet the chances are good that sleep-disordered breathing is an often-overlooked factor in morning headaches of any kind.

Migraines are intense and debilitating headaches that can last for days. According to the National Institutes of Health, about

---

4 Moldofsky, Harvey MD; Scarisbrick, Phillip BS, "Induction of Neurasthenic Musculoskeletal Pain Syndrome by Selective Sleep Stage Deprivation," *Psychosomatic Medicine*, January/February 1976, Volume 38, Issue 1. http://www.ncbi.nlm.nih.gov/pubmed/176677 See also: http://www.sciencedirect.com/science/journal/10870792/5/5 Moldofsky, Harvey, "Sleep and Pain," *Sleep Medicine Reviews*, October 2001, Vol. 5, Issue 5, pp.347-415.

12% of the population suffers from migraines, and women are three times more likely to experience migraines than men.[5] That's about 36 million Americans who suffer from migraines,[6] and they are often unable to work because of the pain. The World Health Organization considers migraines to be among the 20 most debilitating illnesses around the world, and there is no known "cure."[7]

Though it might seem logical that migraines would affect the quality of sleep, it is actually quality of sleep that affects migraines. Most migraines occur during either REM sleep or deep, delta sleep.[8]

Insomnia often goes hand-in-hand with chronic migraines. The SDB causes the brain's panic response, alerting the brain and body to lighter sleep or remain in a waking state. In this way, the reduced oxygen serves as the initial trigger for the insomnia, rather than the migraine itself.

Cluster headaches are rare; they occur mainly in men, but affect less than 1% of the population.[9] The intense pain clusters on one side of the head, often during the night, but may repeat over the course of several days. Cluster headaches typically occur during the first period of REM sleep, about 90 minutes after a person has fallen asleep.[10]

Hypnic headaches are short but intense headaches that tend to happen in the middle of the night, usually at the same time every night, awakening the sleeper. Hypnic headaches have been directly linked to sleep apnea. While hypnic headaches are also rare, they are more common among people over fifty. Hypnic headaches

---

5 Migraine, Medline, National Institutes of Health, November 5, 2013. http://www.nlm.nih.gov/medlineplus/migraine.html

6 "About Migraine," American Migraine Foundation, 2014. http://www.americanmigrainefoundation.org/about-migraine/

7 Ibid.

8 Weintraub, James, DO, Neurologist and Sleep Disorders Specialist, Michigan Head Pain and Neurological Institute, "Sleep Disorders and Headache," posted here: http://www.headache-help.org/sleep-disorders-and-headache

9 http://www.webmd.com/migraines-headaches/guide/cluster-headaches

10 http://www.touchneurology.com/articles/cluster-headache-diagnosis-and-treatment

can also occur during naps.[11] OSA is common among people with hypnic headaches.[12]

SDBs and Headaches

Our patients with headaches experience a reduction in severity and frequency of headaches when their sleep-disordered breathing is treated.

While research results have been mixed, many researchers have found that people with OSA tend to have more headaches than people who have no SDBs. International headache authorities and authors of the textbook *The Headaches* refer to what has been termed a "sleep apnea headache," which occurs only briefly upon awakening. "When the sleep disorder was treated with success, the headache generally disappeared."[13]

TMJ – Temporomandibular Joint Syndrome (Jaw Pain)

Symptoms of TMJ disorders include clicking and popping, jaw pain, ear pain, dizziness and feeling of fullness or ringing in the ear. Airway-centered disorder in adults often leads to clenching and grinding teeth, which in turn often leads to TMJ (jaw) pain, headaches, earaches, as well as back and neck pain.

If you've ever been told you have TMJ or TMD (Temporomandibular Joint Disorder), or if you have pain or clicking and popping sounds in your jaw, then a retruded (or pushed-back) lower jaw is the likely cause of both your pain and your sleep-disordered breathing.

---

11 Swanson, Jerry W., MD, "I am awakened by nighttime headaches. What should I do?" Mayo Clinic Patient Health Care and Information online, February 5, 2014 http://www.mayoclinic.org/diseases-conditions/chronic-daily-headaches/expert-answers/nighttime-headaches/faq-20057919

12 Rains, Jeanetta, PhD, "Sleep and Headache Disorders," Headache: *The Journal of Head and Face Pain,* November 4, 2010, virtual issue: http://www.headachejournal.org/view/0/SleepAndHeadacheDisorders.html

13 Olesen, Jes, et al, *The Headaches, Third Edition,* Lippincott, Williams, & Wilkins, 2005, p. 991.

When your jaw is out-of-alignment, your whole body can get thrown out-of-alignment, contributing to pain anywhere in the body. That pain can start with TMJ.

An estimated 10 million Americans struggle with TMJ.[14] The temporomandibular joint is where the lower and upper jaws meet, directly in front of the ears. The jaw and the muscles work together there, not only for chewing and swallowing, but also for keeping the airway open.

TMJ and sleep-disordered breathing seem to go hand-in-hand with headaches. In our practices, most of the patients coming in with TMJ complaints also have airway issues. Patients referred to us for airway treatment frequently have chronic headaches and neck pain.

Jack had myoclonic spasms when he first came to see Dr Howard Hindin. Dr Hindin states that these myoclonic spasms resulted from Jack's TMJ, because the body can set off the jaw, and the jaw can set off the body. Jack says: "if I haven't worked out in the gym, my muscles tighten up, and then my neck, and then the jaw triggers. Trauma in my childhood led to fear and jaw clenching. Dr Hindin made a biteguard which protected my teeth from clenching. The spasms have been reduced, but I have tried multiple approaches, so what I can say is the mouth appliance has been part of the solution to all of my TMJ issues – the pain, structural problems, and the myoclonic spasms."

Custom-fitting dental appliances to treat sleep-disordered breathing generally improves TMJ symptoms such as clicking and headaches. Treating sleep-disordered breathing with a per-

---

14 Estimated rates of TMJ vary widely, although a higher incidence occurs in women, and surprisingly high rates among young adults, given that it is a condition involving chronic pain. See, for instance: http://onlinelibrary.wiley.com/doi/10.1111/j.1751-9861.2012.00082.x/abstract Doyle, Nicole, Chung-Yi Chiu, et al, "The Prevalence of Temporomandibular Joint and Muscle Disorders in African Americans," *Journal of Applied Biobehavioral Research,* Vol. 17, Issue 4, pages 249-260, December 2012.

"Prevalence of TMJD and Its Signs and Symptoms," National Institute of Dental and Craniofacial Research, National Institutes of Health, http://www.nidcr.nih.gov/datastatistics/finddatabytopic/facialpain/prevalencetmjd.htm

sonally-fitted dental appliance will also help manage bruxism and clenching.

A tight frenum, commonly called a tongue-tie (ankyloglossia), can cause "oro-facial myofunctional disorders" or OMDs, which may complicate treatment of TMJ unless the tongue-tie is released.[15] Tongue-ties can also cause structural changes in the neck and back such as lordosis (sway back) and kyphosis (upper back rounded forward).[16] Because of these structural changes, ankyloglossia may also be the cause of tension and even pain in the jaw, shoulder, head, and neck[17] (please see Dominique's story below). Therefore, a tight frenum must be ruled out as one possible source of pain in dental exams of TMJ patients.

Researchers in India found that ankyloglossia is often associated with poor jaw development and malocclusion.[18] Tongue-tie, whether a classic or even a slight tongue-tie, can cause airway issues and contribute to sleep-disordered breathing as well.[19]

---

15 Fabbie, Paula, RDH, BS, OMT, "The Sleep Team: a team approach is needed for screening patients for orofacial myofunctional disorders," *RDHmag.com*, October 2014, pp. 56-60, 100.

16 Olivi, G, et al, "Lingual Frenectomy: Functional Evaluation and new therapeutical approach," *European Journal of Paediatric Dentistry,* Vol. 13/2, 2012, pp. 101-106.

17 This is an area where more research is needed. All we have is individual case studies, such as Dominique's story. Also, Dr William M. Hang, DDS, posted an interview on *YouTube* of a patient after she had received a frenectomy, in which she speaks of the release of tension, even from her shoulders, as though she had taken a muscle relaxant: https://www.youtube.com/watch?v=Un21c9t5toE

18 Srinivasan, Bhadrinath, and Arun B. Chitharanjan, "Skeletal and Dental Characteristics in Subjects with Ankyloglossia," *Progress in Orthodontics,* 2013, 14:44. http://www.progressinorthodontics.com/content/14/1/44

19 Burkhart, Nancy W., BSDH, EDD, "Ankyloglossia: Are You Paying Attention?" *RDH Magazine* online, Dentistry iQ Network, 2014. Burkhart is an adjunct associate professor in the department of periodontics at Baylor College of Dentistry and the Texas A & M Health Science Center, Dallas. She quotes an OMT on the issue of tongue-ties, TMJ, and airways: Marge Foran, RDH, is a therapist specializing in orofacial myofunctional

We find in our practices that fully half of our patients with TMJ are women in perimenopause (early stages of menopause). Perimenopause is a time when obstructive sleep apnea starts for many women.

Perimenopause, TMJ, migraines, and sleep-disordered breathing are all intertwined. TMJ, sleep-disordered breathing, and perimenopause with its fluctuating estrogen and progesterone levels are all linked to disrupted sleep, which in turn leads to headaches. We have found that when we deal with the airway issue, enabling a woman to sleep at night, the other painful symptoms recede.

Bruxism

As dentists, we see the damage to teeth from bruxism every day. Bruxism includes clenching, bracing, gnashing, and grinding of teeth. Such clenching and grinding is not only very destructive to teeth, but also to overall health. Sleep bruxism is defined as a parasomnia or a stereotyped movement disorder.

OSA is the number one risk factor for bruxism. In fact, one in four people with OSA grind their teeth, according to research from Baylor University.[20] This is especially true in men, who tend to report more sleep apnea and snoring than women.

---

therapy and works with patients who have ankyloglossia in Montana. She made the following comment regarding ankyloglossia:

"Ankyloglossia is one of several contributing factors of orofacial myofunctional disorders. If the lingual frenum is restricted, the limited movement of the tongue may influence the normal growth and development of the oral and nasal cavities and impact muscle patterns and function. This may have many lifelong consequences ranging from difficulty wearing dentures, compensatory speech habits, orthodontic relapse, swallowing disorders, ineffective oral cleansing, and difficulty playing some wind instruments to name a few. A tight lingual frenum has a potential impact on the intrinsic and extrinsic muscles of the tongue.

"In the area of TMD and sleep disordered breathing, it is important to evaluate the lingual frenum. A dysfunctional oral muscle patterning of the tongue and orofacial muscles may influence these disorders or conditions. At any age, it is recommended that a consult occur with an orofacial myofunctional therapist prior to a surgical procedure."

20 http://www.sciencedaily.com/releases/2009/11/091102171213.htm

Sleep bruxism has been found to occur during all stages of sleep, but is usually associated with moving from a deeper to a lighter stage of sleep including both light and deep stages of non-REM sleep, as well as REM sleep, most often following a microarousal.[21] Researchers in Japan did find that episodes of sleep bruxism reduce the amount of slow-wave (deep) sleep.[22]

Patricia, age 55, had her jaw go out of socket 12 years ago, and an orthodontist treated her with a nightguard. About 4 years ago, she was in a car accident that caused facial impact on the steering wheel, leaving her with slight nerve damage. She had ringing in her left ear and headaches. Her jaw started popping out in December 2013, so she came to see Dr Michael Gelb in February of 2014. Dr Gelb fitted her with an appliance that brought her jaw back to center, and decompressed the left side. After two months, Patricia has "no pain, no ringing, and no excessive daytime sleepiness." She is "sleeping better."

Bruxism can result in tooth pain, TMJ pain, and headaches. So bruxism directly contributes to that vicious cycle of chronic pain, poor sleep, and poor health.

Misfiring neurochemistry, a malfunctioning autonomic nervous system, sleep-disordered breathing, and sleep arousals all have been cited as potential causes for bruxism, but researchers have not pinpointed the exact reasons why some people "brux." What we have found in our practices is that, if you are bruxing, you very likely have an airway issue. Bruxism may be the body's attempt to reopen the airway.

Experts once believed that bruxing served to release the day's stress. Historically, dentists were taught that people clenched their jaws because their teeth didn't fit together well. Most dentists then

21 Bader,Gaby, and Gilles Lavigne, "Sleep Bruxism; an overview of an oromandibular sleep movement disorder," *Sleep Medicine Review,* Vol. 4, Issue 1, pp. 27-43, February 2000. http://www.smrv-journal.com/article/S1087-0792(99)90070-9/abstract

22 Huynh, N, et al, "Sleep Bruxism Is Associated to Micro-Arousals and an increase in cardiac sympathetic activity," *Journal of Sleep Research,* 2006, 15:339-346. http://onlinelibrary.wiley.com/doi/10.1111/j.1365-2869.2006.00536.x/pdf

did what they therefore believed was best: they shaved down the teeth.

When teeth are ground down, the size of the mouth is decreased, bringing the roof and the floor of the mouth closer together. This reduces the airway. As little as a millimeter in height results in an even greater loss in volume in your upper airway, affecting how you breathe and how you feel. If you like breathing easily, do not allow your dentist to grind down your teeth.

Bruxism Triad

Many patients experience a "bruxism triad": arousal-induced tooth grinding, airway-associated sleep-related disturbances and sleep-related gastroesophageal reflux (GERD or heartburn). It is not entirely clear why these three conditions cluster together, but it *is* obvious that this triad works against you to interrupt sleep and create pain throughout your body.

According to Dr Jeffrey Rouse, DDS, of the people who suffer from sleep bruxism, at least one-third also have sleep-disordered breathing conditions, including sleep apnea, periodic leg movement during sleep, and headaches.[23] Researchers know that as sleep-related disturbances increase, so does the amount of bruxing. Almost 50% of people with upper airway resistance syndrome complain of bruxism,[24] and remember, obstructive sleep apnea is the highest risk factor for tooth grinding during sleep. The Baylor study also found that 35% of those with obstructive sleep apnea complained of nighttime heartburn and GERD.[25]

Tooth wear is one way dentists detect bruxism. Tooth wear means the tooth has lost its basic structure because of:

- Attrition (loss of tooth structure because of contact with opposite teeth),

---

23 Rouse, Jeffrey S., DDS, "The Bruxism Triad: Sleep bruxism, sleep disturbance, and sleep-related GERD," *Inside Dentistry,* May 2010, pp. 32-44. http://www.tcbsc.net/pdfs/Inside%20Dentistry%20-%20Article%20 -%20Bruxism%20Triad%201.pdf

24 Ibid.

25 http://www.sciencedaily.com/releases/2009/11/091102171213.htm

- Abrasion (scratching from toothbrushes, toothpicks or floss), and/or
- Erosion (caused by acids, including stomach acid from GERD, wearing away the tooth enamel).

As you can see, both bruxism and GERD contribute to tooth wear, which can also be painful. Since pain disrupts sleep as well as interferes with activities during the day, tooth wear from bruxism and GERD becomes part of that vicious circle of sleep disturbance, inflammation and increased pain.

However, excessive tooth wear does not occur simply from the friction of clenching and grinding teeth against teeth; it's also a matter of saliva. Saliva is a lubricant, so it can reduce the friction and the damage to the teeth; yet, less saliva is produced at night, which makes sleep bruxing more damaging.

Changes in body position and pressure changes in the esophagus resulting from sleep-disordered breathing often allows acid from the digestive tract to move up the esophagus, setting the stage for acid reflux (GERD) at night.[26] During sleep, acid may even pool in the mouth, and thus play a role in tooth destruction.

Left untreated, bruxism can lead to excessive tooth wear and decay, periodontal tissue damage, as well as TMJ and headaches, among other painful outcomes. If you have sleep bruxism, we especially recommend that you get a sleep study and see an Airway Centric® dentist to have your airway evaluated. You can be fitted with appliances that can help reduce or eliminate most of the problems associated with bruxism.

Actions for Reducing Pain

Sleep is #1: Get more sleep and follow a good pattern of sleep hygiene. Researchers at the University of North Carolina found that women with chronic migraines experienced a significant reduction in the frequency and intensity of migraines by following healthy sleep habits.

---

26 Demeter, Pal and Akos Pap, "The relationship between gastroesophageal reflux disease and obstructive sleep apnea," *Journal of Gastroenterology,* September 2004, Volume 39, Issue 9, pp. 815-820. http://link.springer.com/article/10.1007/s00535-004-1416-8

"Their instructions were to go to bed at the same time every night, at a time that allows for eight hours' time in bed; eliminate TV watching, reading or listening to music while in bed; use visualization techniques to shorten the amount of time it took them to fall asleep; eat supper at least four hours before going to bed and limit fluid intake within two hours of bedtime; and do not take naps."[27]

» **Action: Get a sleep study.** Even if you think you "just" have a headache, or "just" have joint pain, or "just" clench and grind or brux your teeth, a sleep study can show whether or not you also have an underlying airway issue. Treating the airway issue so that you sleep well at night may significantly lessen your pain.

» **Action: Eat less sugar.** According to the *Harvard Medical School Family Health Guide*, highly refined foods as well as foods high in carbohydrates tend to raise blood sugar levels too fast and too high, causing the body to increase levels of cytokines, contributing to increased overall inflammation in the body.[28]

» **Action: Seek appliance therapy.** While most of dentistry from 1925 to the present involved moving the jaw back, Dr Harold Gelb, D.M.D, saw the logic of bringing the jaw *forward* into a natural decompressed joint position, which just happens to be an open airway posture. Dr Harold Gelb created the Gelb appliance, which alleviated most TMJ problems and serendipitously opened closed airways at night through mandibular orthopedic repositioning of the jaw (bringing the jaw forward).

The Gelb, Farrar and functional orthodontic appliances all brought the jaws forward and created healthier looking faces

---

27 Crayton, Stephanie, "Improving sleep behaviors reduces frequency and intensity of headaches," The University of North Carolina at Chapel Hill, news release, June 23, 2006. http://www.unc.edu/news/archives/jun06/migraine062206.htm

28 "What you eat can fuel or cool inflammation, a key driver of heart disease, diabetes, and other chronic conditions," Harvard Medical School Family Health Guide, February 2007, http://www.health.harvard.edu/fhg/updates/What-you-eat-can-fuel-or-cool-inflammation-a-key-driver-of-heart-disease-diabetes-and-other-chronic-conditions.shtml

while promoting better sleep. Today, we often use modified Gelb appliances during the day (the legacy of co-author Dr Michael Gelb's father). We use a number of different oral appliances at night to maintain an open airway and promote healthier, more restful sleep.

We recommend that you consult with a dentist who is able to custom-fit you for an appliance that not only reduces bruxism and re-aligns your jaw to reduce the pain of TMJ, but also will enable you to maintain an open airway while you sleep.

Part III- No Peak Performance Without the Breath of Life

10

CHAPTER

Mental and Physical Daily Performance

Here's a story about our good friend and colleague, Dr Jay, who tore both of his rotator cuffs in a bout of overenthusiasm—he was 59 when this happened. The injury forced him to retire from racquetball, his passion and favorite pastime. A year later, he had put on 40 pounds due to lack of exercise. His blood pressure shot up and he burst a blood vessel in his eye. We warned Dr Jay he was a great candidate for a heart attack or a stroke.

He finally confessed to us that he had developed a bad habit on his way to work: He would pull up to a red light and put his car in park and fall asleep until the honking woke him and the cycle began again at the next red light. We convinced him to do a sleep study. Sure enough, our suspicions were confirmed: Dr Jay had sleep-disordered breathing (SBD).

He was good as new—or almost—after we fitted him with a nighttime appliance and CPAP machine. Feeling better gave him the initiative to have surgery on his rotator cuffs and today he's lost the weight and is back on the racquetball court and even occasionally manages to win a game or two from us.

The High Cost of Less Sleep

Many people drive while sleepy, just as our friend Dr Jay used to do. There are obviously many risks both to driving and to working while sleepy. Whether a person is sleepy because of a lack of sleep, because of sleep-disordered breathing, or because of insomnia or working night shifts, the consequences can literally be deadly.

The 2013 New York train wreck in which four people died was caused by the train engineer falling asleep. The engineer suffered from excessive daytime sleepiness resulting from a severe case of obstructive sleep apnea.

Researchers at the Institute of Medicine report that some of the most dangerous and environmentally devastating events in recent history have been caused by sleep disorders, shift work, or lack of sleep. Specifically, loss of sleep and night-shift related errors contributed to:

- The meltdown of the nuclear reactor at Chernobyl
- The meltdown of the nuclear reactor at Three Mile Island
- The tragic explosion at the Bhopal, India, chemical plant
- The grounding of the Exxon Valdez oil tanker
- The grounding of the Star Princess cruise ship[1]

According to the Centers for Disease Control, "Driving while drowsy causes an estimated 1,550 fatalities annually, as well as 40,000 non-fatal injuries each year in the United States."[2] Driving with just one night of sleep deprivation is the equivalent of driving drunk.[3]

Due to public safety risks, some employers—like the military, NASA, and the airlines—are required to test employees' wakeful-

---

1 Colten, Harvey R, and BM Altevogt, *Sleep Disorders and Sleep Deprivation: An Unmet Public Health Problem,* (Washington, DC: National Academies Press), 2006, Ch. 4. http://www.ncbi.nlm.nih.gov/books/NBK19958/

2 Morbidity and Mortality Weekly Report, Weekly / Vol. 60 / No. 8 March 4, 2011. "Unhealthy Sleep-Related Behaviors — 12 States, 2009." http://www.cdc.gov/mmwr/PDF/wk/mm6008.pdf

3 http://drowsydriving.org/about/detection-and-prevention/

ness. As the incidence of sleep apnea rises, such testing becomes more critical.

For example, the 2013 New York City train wreck, in which four people died, occurred after the train engineer fell asleep. The cause: excessive daytime sleepiness resulting from a severe case of obstructive sleep apnea.[4] As a matter of fact, the National Transportation Safety Board's official ruling was that the accident was caused by the engineer's untreated obstructive sleep apnea.[5] In other words, the accident could have been prevented—and lives saved—if the engineer's sleep apnea had been diagnosed and treated.

Potentially helpful to employers for both workplace safety and public safety, testing has been developed to measure quickly and effectively an individual's ability to function well and alertly. Dr David Dinges of the University of Pennsylvania developed the 10-minute Psychomotor Vigilance Test (PVT), and has now even developed a 3-minute version (the PVT-B), that can easily be used to test a worker's attention and reaction time.. Both tests have been shown to be reliable in demonstrating whether or not a person is suffering from sleep deprivation.[6]

Workers themselves experience increased risks due to loss of sleep. Researchers in Switzerland found that workers with sleep problems were 62% more likely to experience workplace injuries, and that 13% of workplace injuries occurred because of employee sleep problems.[7] In a twenty-year-long study of almost 50,000

---

4 "Train driver in deadly New York crash had 'severe' sleep disorder, NTSB says," Associated Press in White Plains, NY, theguardian.com, Monday 7 April, 2014, 15:39 EDT http://www.theguardian.com/world/2014/apr/07/new-york-train-crash-william-rockefeller-ntsb-report

5 http://blogs.rollcall.com/the-container/ntsb-cites-sleep-apnea-in-fatal-train-accident/?dcz=

6 Dinges, David F, Mathias Basner, and Daniel Mollicone, "Validity and sensitivity of a brief psychomotor vigilance test (PVT-B) to total and partial sleep deprivation," *Acta Astronautica,* 69 (2011) 949-959. Accessed here on November 22, 2014: https://www.med.upenn.edu/uep/user_documents/Basner2011-ValidityandsensitivityofabriefPVT.pdf

7 Uehli, Katrin, et al, "Sleep problems and work injuries: a systematic review and meta-analysis," *Sleep Medicine Reviews,* Vol. 18, Issue 1,

people in Sweden, researchers found that people who reported disrupted sleep were almost twice as likely to die in workplace accidents.[8]

Medically-related deaths and errors of diagnosis and treatment in hospitals are also increased by sleep loss. According to The Institute of Medicine, research has shown that residents working more than 80 hours a week were 50% more likely to report making a serious medical error that led to an adverse patient outcome than those who worked less than 80 hours per week.

Moreover, a study that reduced the number of hours some interns worked and compared their error rates to those of interns on a traditional schedule found that the rate of serious medical errors was 22% higher among those who worked the longer traditional hours. Because of the randomized controls in the study, the difference can largely be explained by the fact that those who worked fewer hours were able to sleep an average of about six hours more per week.[9]

When we consider the high rates of undiagnosed SDBs, the potential risks and costs to society become more dramatically apparent. According to the American Academy of Sleep Medicine, about 80% to 90% of adults with OSA remain undiagnosed[10]—and that's just sleep apnea, not all the other forms of SDBs that take a toll on people's lives and health, along with their ability to concentrate and stay alert.

Performance at Work

We're a nation of multi-taskers: answering an urgent e-mail in the midst of a conference call, writing a memo while eating a quick lunch desk-side, taking a call from the boss while driving or juggling

---

February 2014, pages 61-73. http://www.sciencedirect.com/science/article/pii/S1087079213000087

8 Colten and Altevogt, http://www.ncbi.nlm.nih.gov/books/NBK19958/

9 Ibid.

10 American Academy of Sleep Medicine's 2008 fact sheet, "Obstructive Sleep Apnea," available online: http://www.aasmnet.org/resources/factsheets/sleepapnea.pdf

three or four requests from employers or employees. And that's just at the office.

Outside the office, "thanks" to rampant connectivity, we field "quick" questions via email, text and phone while standing on the sidelines of the kids' soccer game. Then there are independent workers with home offices who are equally challenged when it comes to down time because their work life blends seamlessly with household responsibilities.

In today's work world, those long hours are expected of us. The boss wants a team player, a productive worker with a steady upbeat mood, a winning personality.

Yet, having a sleep disorder such as obstructive sleep apnea (OSA) can manifest as irritability and inability to concentrate. Children with sleep problems have trouble focusing, seem socially withdrawn or aggressive, and often cannot work at their highest capabilities. Adults who have sleep disorders experience similar side-effects, and these often manifest themselves in the workplace, hampering reasoning and decision-making. (MRI results have demonstrated which areas of the brain fail to become activated during a verbal learning task undertaken in a state of sleep deprivation.[11])

Researchers at the University of Oxford found that people with problems sleeping experienced shrinkage in three parts of the brain: the frontal, temporal, and parietal lobes. The study noted an

> **Louis, a middle-aged TV executive,** had been diagnosed with a severe case of sleep apnea and a small airway. He used to snore and wake himself up. Louis was not interested in a CPAP machine, so he came to see Dr Michael Gelb to be fitted with a sleep appliance. After a few months of using the nighttime appliance, Louis reports that he is sleeping well, and also performing better during the daytime.

---

11 Durmer, Jeffrey S, MD, PhD, and David F. Dinges, PhD, "Neurocognitive Consequences of Sleep Deprivation," *Seminars in Neurology,* Volume 25, Number 1, 2005. https://www.med.upenn.edu/uep/user_documents/dfd3.pdf

association but it has not been determined which one causes the other, or if causality works both ways.[12]

Another study found that the brains of people who get less sleep age faster too. According to European researchers who measured the size of the ventricles in the brain, people with poor sleep quality experienced greater loss of gray matter over a period of three-and-a-half years, regardless of age, although people over 60 experienced even greater losses.[13]

It's estimated that sleepiness costs billions of dollars annually in lost worker productivity. Reducing nighttime sleep by as little as 1.5 hours for just one night could mean a 32% drop in daytime alertness.[14] With so much to do, no one can afford to miss even a little sleep.

A study by Dr Clelia Lima and Dr Elizabeth Rash at the College of Nursing at the University of Central Florida found a significant cost-benefit for companies that screened employees for OSA and offered CPAP therapy. They based their research on studies showing that OSA can reduce work productivity by 30%. Their conclusion is that large corporations can save millions of dollars annually by screening their employees for OSA and providing treatment, even if only 75% of the employees are compliant in using the CPAP machine.[15]

---

12 Almendrala, Anna, "The Frightening Connection Between Lack of Sleep and A Shrinking Brain," HuffPost *Healthy Living,* September 4, 2010. http://www.huffingtonpost.com/2014/09/04/sleep-shrinking-brain_n_5739442.html?utm_hp_ref=healthy-living&ir=Healthy+Living

13 Willingham, Val, "Lack of sleep may shrink your brain," *cnn.com*, Sept. 4, 2014. http://www.cnn.com/2014/09/04/health/no-sleep-brain-size/

14 Bonnet, Michael H. and Donna L. Arand, "We Are Chronically Sleep Deprived," *Sleep*, 18(10):908-911, 1995. http://web.arizona.edu/~vas/478/weare.pdf Also cited here: http://www.webmd.com/sleep-disorders/features/important-sleep-habits

15 Dusik, Doug, "Screening high-risk employees for sleep apnea could save a corporation millions of dollars," Sleep 2011 Media Relations, June 2, 2011; research presented by Dr Clelia Lima and Dr Elizabeth M. Rash at the Sleep 2011, 25th Anniversary Meeting of the Associated Professional Sleep Societies. http://www.aasmnet.org/articles.aspx?id=2309

A study published in the journal *Sleep* shows that workers with OSA were almost 14 times more likely to have had job-performance problems, including falling asleep on the job or missing a day's work, during just a four-week period. People with OSA and excessive daytime sleepiness were almost four times as likely to have had a pay cut or miss out on a promotion.[16]

A Finnish study looked at how likely both men and women are to miss workdays before they are diagnosed with sleep apnea. Men are 60% more likely to miss work, and women are 80% more likely to miss work when suffering from undiagnosed and untreated OSA than people who do not have sleep apnea.[17]

Sexual Performance

It's no surprise that without deep, restful sleep, women do not become easily aroused, and men's sexual performance lags. However, the lack of interest in sex resulting from poor sleep goes far beyond the simple, "Honey, I'm too tired tonight."

One aspect of sleep that leads to morning erections is REM sleep. If a man wakes up with an erection, it is likely that he is awakening from REM sleep. During REM sleep, the parasympathetic nervous system triggers the tissues of the penis to be filled with blood, thus becoming firm. Waking up with an erection is a good sign that a man is both obtaining REM sleep and has no physiological basis for erectile dysfunction.[18] So, adequate sleep is essential for the full expression of sexual potential.

---

16 Omachi, Theodore A, MD, MBA, et al, "Obstructive Sleep Apnea: A Risk Factor for Work Disability," *Sleep*, Volume 32, Issue 6, pp. 791-798, 2009. http://www.journalsleep.org/ViewAbstract.aspx?pid=27478

17 Sjosten, Noora, PhD, et al, "Increased Risk of Lost Work Days Prior to the Diagnosis of Sleep Apnea," *Chest*, 2009, 136(1):130-136. http://journal.publications.chestnet.org/article.aspx?articleid=1089906&issueno=1

18 Peters, Brandon, MD, "Does a Lack of Morning Wood Suggest Erectile Dysfunction?" *About Health*, November 17, 2014, about.com. Accessed here on November 22, 2014: http://sleepdisorders.about.com/od/sleepandgeneralhealth/f/Does-A-Lack-Of-Morning-Wood-Suggest-Erectile-Dysfunction.htm

Sexual performance in both men and women also clearly depends on a healthy blood flow to the genitals. Increased blood flow to the penis causes engorgement so the penis swells. The primary trigger for increased blood flow to both the penis and the clitoris is nitric oxide, a powerful vasodilator that is naturally produced in the human body. Some of the most popular drug treatments for erectile dysfunction work by increasing the production of nitric oxide.

> **There's an established association** between sleep apnea and sexual performance. For those men in the study who regularly used CPAP over a three-month period, overall sexual satisfaction improved 88.3%.

Proper nasal breathing (as opposed to mouth breathing) stimulates the release of nitric oxide. The brain also produces nitric oxide, but that production can be decreased by OSA. Some researchers found that men with sleep apnea have lower levels of nitric oxide, and when they use a CPAP machine during sleep, their levels of nitric oxide increase.[19]

It makes sense that reproduction is very low on the brain's priority list when survival is at stake. Why try to procreate if you might not live another day—or hour? Arousal becomes physiologically unimportant when the body is struggling merely to get enough air.

Sleep deprivation can cause reduced sex drives as well. Testosterone and other sex hormones rise when the body is rested and fall when it is not.[20]

A German study linking sexual dysfunction in men to OSA found that men with OSA who use CPAP machines long term (an average of three years) have dramatic improvements in their sexual abilities,

---

19 Ip, Mary S.M., et al, "Circulating Nitric Oxide Is Suppressed in Obstructive Sleep Apnea and Is Reversed by Nasal Continuous Positive Airway Pressure," *American Journal of Respiratory and Critical Care Medicine,* Volume 162, Issue 6, December 2000. http://www.atsjournals. org/doi/abs/10.1164/ajrccm.162.6.2002126#.VGEuZ_IdUod

20 See for instance: http://www.everydayhealth.com/low-testosterone/ low-testosterone-and-sleep-deprivation-whats-the-link.aspx

demonstrating the potential for treatment of OSA to reverse sexual dysfunction.[21]

A US-based study at Walter Reed National Military Medical Hospital looked at the effect of CPAP treatment on the sexual satisfaction of young to middle-aged men (average age: 45). Those who reported erectile dysfunction experienced significant improvements in ED. For those men in the study who regularly used CPAP over a three-month period, overall sexual satisfaction improved 88.3%. The men experienced 71.7% improvement in erectile dysfunction overall, and "normalization" of erectile function in 41.2%. Even those who did not initially report problems with ED experienced enhancement of their sexual performance when regularly using a CPAP machine.[22]

When working with our patients, we often find a link between ED and sleep apnea. In fact, one smart patient concluded that if he woke up with an erection, his sleep apnea treatment was working.

Actions to Improve Performance

» **Action: Monitor snoring.** If your partner snores or says you do, ask your doctor for a sleep study, and see an Airway Centric® dentist.

» **Action: Monitor morning alertness.** If you're hitting the snooze button three or four times and dragging yourself out of bed, fortifying yourself with coffee and struggling to get to work on time, you're either staying up too late or you have SDB. Again, ask your doctor for a sleep study. Other signs you may have sleep-disordered breathing and should have airway and sleep evaluations:

---

21 Budweiser, Stephan, et al, "Long term changes of sexual function in men with obstructive sleep apnea after initiation of continuous positive airway pressure," *Journal of Sexual Medicine*, February 2013, 10(2):524-31. http://www.pubfacts.com/detail/23088487/Long-term-changes-of-sexual-function-in-men-with-obstructive-sleep-apnea-after-initiation-of-continu

22 "CPAP Use Improves Sexual Function in Younger Men," Department of Defense, US Medicine, *The Voice of Federal Medicine,* August 2012. http://www.usmedicine.com/agencies/department-of-defense-dod/cpap-use-improves-sexual-function-in-younger-men/

- On-the job-accidents
- Employer critical of job performance
- Difficulty managing anger and frustration on the job
- Declining athletic performance
- Inability to find the energy to exercise
- Falling grades in school
- Loss of libido (interest in sex) in both men and women, erectile dysfunction in men, inability to reach orgasm in women

» **Action: Consider a CPAP machine or an oral appliance to open your airway.**

11

C H A P T E R

Airways and Athletic Performance

Dominique, age 28, loves to stay in shape through CrossFit training. For years, she never understood why she had pain traveling down her neck and into her trapezius muscles, especially burning pain in her shoulders after CrossFit workouts. She thought maybe this was normal. Dominique also suffered from severe pain under her ears and under her eyes. She thought it must be from sinuses, but she found out she had no sinus infection. The pain got worse, so she went to an oral surgeon, who gave her a prescription for pain medication, and made her a nighttime appliance, but it didn't help.

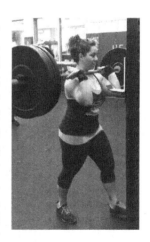

She came to see Dr Gelb. He made her a daytime appliance and a night guard, and told her to "be an advocate for yourself" and "find the root of the problem." The pain lessened, but did not go away. Dr Gelb recommended that Dominique see Paula Fabbie,

OMT, who told her she was "tongue-tied" and needed a frenectomy, or frenulum release.

Dominique saw an oral surgeon who told her she might need jaw surgery, which scared her. So, again she called Paula, who reassured her that all she needed was a frenectomy. Dominique had her tongue released surgically.

The next day, Dominique awoke and realized she had no pain, no headache. She felt free, as though "the rubber band that had had my neck in a bind had snapped."

Dominique never thought anything was wrong with her sleeping, but now she felt good when she woke up, and for the first time in her life, she had (or remembered) a dream. The burning in her shoulders was gone; the agitation (anxiety) she used to feel was gone. She said, "I no longer feel on edge."

She continued working with Paula Fabbie doing oro-facial my-ofunctional therapy exercises, which are beneficial, especially for speech, after a frenulum release. Months later, Dominique wrote:

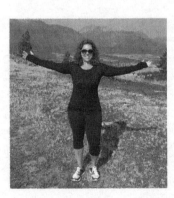

"After the tongue-tie release, I felt an instant release in my shoulders. Since February, I have not felt the intense pain I felt on a daily basis after working out. My workouts continue to improve. In CrossFit, we have what we call Personal Records, which is a goal you strive to achieve every few weeks to see how your strength has improved. I'm proud to say my numbers keep increasing and I know for a fact it is because of the tongue-tie release.

"I sleep better and my muscles are able to heal better. As a result, I'm gaining more mental and physical strength than ever before. My headaches have eased dramatically. The chiropractor I see at least 3 times a month notices a drastic difference in my neck muscles since the tongue-tie release. I have a positive outlook on life and I am overall a happier person.

"I am feeling fantastic! I feel healthy and I wake up ready to start each morning with a positive outlook. I have less anxiety and I'm a more peaceful person than I have ever been. I was recently offered a teaching job and am beyond thrilled to begin my dream profession."

As Dominique's story reveals, even at younger ages, having an airway issue of any sort can reduce our athletic ability. Improving that airway issue, even if it requires the time, effort and cost of an interdisciplinary approach—as it did in Dominique's case— can improve both one's athletic abilities and recovery time from workouts, not to mention general quality of life.

> **Stanford swimmers who slept more** swam a 15 meter sprint 0.51 seconds faster, started 0.15 seconds faster off the blocks, and even improved their turns by 0.10 seconds. Many of them not only achieved personal bests, but also broke records held both at Stanford, as well as across America.

If you are middle-aged or older, and are lucky enough to have made it this far in life without chronic disease, sexual dysfunction or mood disorders, and your biggest concern is how to keep your body healthy and active, you may still benefit from better breathing.

As we age, many of us see our athletic performance slipping: we can't run as far or as fast; our tennis game isn't as accurate as it once was. Perhaps you satisfy yourself by reliving the glory days of your youth. Perhaps you chalk-up your declining athletic abilities to a demanding sedentary job, to being busy with family obligations, to the weight you've gained since high school, or simply to your age.

Those might all be factors—or not. Sleep plays a pivotal role in everything we do. Most of us don't sleep enough and when we do sleep, we may experience fragmented sleep because of airway obstructions. This could be a factor in waning athletic prowess as we age. It was for our friend Dr Jay from the previous chapter. In fact, the importance of sleep to athletic performance was amply demonstrated in studies of Stanford University athletes.

One of the studies looked at the performance of varsity basketball players. Most of them were mildly sleep deprived averaging about 6.75 hours of sleep at night. They were asked to sleep 10 hours each night. While none succeeded in sleeping that much, they were able to stretch out their z-time to 8.5 hours per night over about a six-week period.

According to researcher Cheri Mah of the Stanford Sleep Disorders Clinic, after achieving this additional sleep time for six weeks, these basketball players sprinted faster (0.7 second improvement) and they improved the accuracy of both their free throws and three-point shots by 9%.[1]

Increased sleep yielded impressive results for other Stanford athletes in additional studies by Mah as well. Stanford swimmers who slept more swam a 15 meter sprint 0.51 seconds faster, started 0.15 seconds faster off the blocks, and even improved their turns by 0.10 seconds. Many of them not only achieved personal bests, but also broke records held both at Stanford, as well as across America. Mah reports similar results have occurred as she has worked with Stanford athletes in various sports: football, tennis, track and field, golf, and cross-country.[2] Mah and her team didn't look into other aspects of the players' lives, but we are willing to bet that their academic performance also improved.

A study at the University of Chicago investigated the same issue from a different angle. Sleep researcher Eve Van Cauter looked at men who were deprived of sleep and found they metabolized glucose less efficiently, and their levels of the stress hormone cortisol were higher.

Van Cauter said that after just a week of sleep restriction, these men—ages 18 to 27 years—experienced a degraded ability to

---

1 Mah CD; Mah KE; Kezirian EJ; Dement WC. The effects of sleep extension on the athletic performance of collegiate basketball players. SLEEP 2011;34(7):943-950. http://www.journalsleep.org/ViewAbstract. aspx?pid=28194

2 American Academy of Sleep Medicine, "Extra Sleep Improves Athletic Performance," ScienceDaily, June 10, 2008. http://www.sciencedaily.com/ releases/2008/06/080609071106.htm

process glucose. Rather than processing it as healthy men should, their ability was similar to what is expected in elderly people.[3]

This study shows that sleep deprivation takes a toll on body processes that are critical for peak athletic performance: glucose metabolism and cortisol status. Glucose is the fuel for athletes, especially for endurance sports. Cortisol interferes with the body's ability to recover from athletic exertion, so sleep loss can increase the likelihood of over-training leading to injury.[4]

Athletic Performance and Airway Issues

If you spend hours in front of a computer every day, you may find yourself hunched forward all day and thinking that your posture comes from fatigue, a sedentary job, or a lack of self-discipline for sitting up straight. In fact, a hunched back and a forward head posture are quite likely the result of an airway obstruction, which forces your body to work harder to breathe, and this can lead to thrusting the head forward to open the airway. With an airway obstruction that leads to sleep-disordered-breathing, it becomes more difficult to stand or sit up straight. If you snore or have sleep apnea or other forms of sleep-disordered breathing (SDB), you awaken unrefreshed, so it can be difficult to find the energy to engage in the sports you love.

The stress on the body from trying so hard to get oxygen leads to tighter muscles, so their range of motion gets limited. Even if you do find the energy to play golf, you may not realize that you don't have the fullest swing possible. In tennis, your backhand has lost its oomph. When you ski, your balance is off. OSA drags down the physical endurance and coordination that athletes need to win.

A study by Dr Marc L. Benton of the Atlantic Sleep and Pulmonary Associates shows that golfers with obstructive sleep apnea who received nasal positive airway pressure (NPAP) improved their

---

3 Quinn, Elizabeth, "Sleep Deprivation and Athletes," About.com, October 28, 2014. http://sportsmedicine.about.com/cs/conditioning/a/aa062800a.htm citing: Spiegel, Karine, et al, "Impact of Sleep Debt on metabolic and endocrine function," The Lancet, Volume 354, Issue 9188, pages 1435-39.

4 Ibid.

daytime sleepiness score and lowered their golf handicaps by as much as three strokes.[5]

When we use Airway Centric® oral appliances to bring athletes' jaws forward to open their airways, their posture improves, their balance steadies and their athletic performance increases. In fact, we witness immediate effects in our offices when an appliance is fitted appropriately for an individual, because we often use muscle testing to determine the best position for a person's jaw. Muscle testing provides an indicator of an open airway and overall muscle strength.

> **When Michael Jordan** stuck out his tongue to make winning shots time-after-time in the last seconds of games, he was intuitively placing his jaw in the Airway Centric® appliance position.

We also find that when an appliance is fitted correctly, a person's heart rate decreases, their balance improves, and they feel a sense of physiological calm. When a patient is fitted for an appliance, if they experience a profound relaxation of the muscles, this indicates the appliance is fitted correctly. When that profound sense of calm is attained, we know we have placed the jaw in the best possible position for opening the airway and decreasing tension.

Breathing properly promotes a sense of calm that's essential for precision sports. Basketball players who remain calm at the free throw line can make the game-winning shot. For tennis players, remaining calm enables the ball coming at you to seem big and slow, so it is very easy to hit with precision. Remaining calm enables longer reaction times and more accurate decision-making.

For instance, military sharp-shooters learn precision and subtlety, which requires not only a state of mental calm but also complete physiological calm. These sharp-shooters actually know how to pull the trigger between heartbeats. As a result, they learn to slow their breath down to slow their heart rate, allowing a longer window to take the shot. Special Forces personnel train to keep their nervous systems in a balanced state, to allow them to stay

---

5 American College of Chest Physicians. (2009, November 5). "Sleep Apnea Improves Golf Game." *ScienceDaily*. Retrieved November 19, 2014 from http://www.sciencedaily.com/releases/2009/11/091102171211.htm

clear-headed, focused, emotionally balanced and physically strong. This is only possible with an open airway.

Bringing the jaw forward to the Gelb 4/7 position opens the airway naturally and enhances health, overall appearance, and athletic performance. This represents a significant shift in the practice of dentistry and orthodontics. From 1930 to 1995, the predominant view was that the jaw was meant to be retruded in order to "fix the bite." This placed the lower jaw backwards, in the old Centric Relation position, which also closed the airway.[6]

When Michael Jordan stuck out his tongue to make winning shots time-after-time in the last seconds of games, he was placing his jaw in the Airway Centric® appliance position. Jordan was intuitively and subconsciously positioning his jaw in a location that allowed him to enter "the zone." This position allows for more oxygen and strength while increasing balance and flexibility.

David Wright of the Mets holds his jaw in this position—with his tongue sticking out—every time he hits a home run; this cannot be a coincidence. Tennis greats Pete Sampras and John McEnroe did the same thing, intuitively and subconsciously.

The practice of using oral appliances to improve athletic performance goes back to the 1970s, starting with the work of John Stenger, dentist for the Notre Dame football team. Dr Stenger and his colleagues did early research on using dental appliances, or mouth guards, to improve athletic performance, improve posture, and release cervical tension. Unfortunately, much of the early research lacked scientific rigor in the design of the experiments. As Dr Harold Gelb (father of author Michael Gelb) reports, the early research was debunked by other research that also lacked scientific rigor.[7]

In actuality, the practice of using a bite splint has a long track record, including for athletic performance and reduction of stress

6 Gelb, Michael, DDS, MS, "Airway Centric®TMJ Philosophy," *California Dental Association Journal,* Volume 42, Number 8, August 2014, pp. 551-562.

7 Gelb, Harold, BS, DMD, "The Relationship Between Jaw Posture and Muscular Strength in Sports Dentistry: A Reappraisal," *The Journal of Craniomandibular Practice,* October 1996, Volume 14, Number 4, pp. 320-325.

and pain. Dr Mark Roettger reports that ancient Roman athletes used leather straps between their teeth to improve their prowess in battle. He also notes that Native American women would ease the pain and stress of childbirth by biting on sticks during delivery. Roettger says that the practice of "biting the bullet" stems from the Civil War, when many amputations were performed without anesthesia; soldiers literally bit on bullets to manage the pain and stress of amputation.[8]

Indeed, one of the early studies on athletic performance and dental appliances was performed by Dr RS Kaufman, who created bite splints for the 1980 U.S. Olympic bobsled team, which resulted in significant decreases in pain and headaches during and after the run for several of the athletes. In addition, some athletes reported greater strength when pushing off at the start of the run.[9]

A follow-up double-blind study with football players used a MORA, or mandibular orthopedic repositioning appliance. The MORA repositions the jaw in a forward position that opens the airway. Results of this study showed that the MORA reduced the number and severity of injuries, especially knee injuries, while also increasing strength.[10]

Later studies found conflicting results; however, Dr Harold Gelb reports that it is the positioning of the jaw with the appliance, not the appliance itself, that makes a difference. Therefore many studies failed to show results, because the appliances were not used to position the jaw properly.[11] Knowing where to position the jaw often was and still is the issue, because dentists haven't been trained to bring the jaw forward into an Airway Centric® position.

As long as dentists favor the position called "Centric Relation," the optimal positioning of the jaw remains an issue when creating bite or mouth guards for athletes.

---

8 Roettger, Mark, DDS, "Performance Enhancement and Oral Appliances," *Aegis Communications,* July/August 2009, Volume 30, Issue 2. https://www.dentalaegis.com/special-issues/2009/08/performance-enhancement-and-oral-appliances

9 Gelb, Harold.

10 Ibid.

11 Ibid.

Derrick Dockery of the Washington Redskins uses a neuro-muscular mouth guard. He misplaced it for a few games. According to *USA Today*, Dockery stated, "I got more winded the games I didn't have it in compared to the games I did have it. My breathing felt different when I wore it. It seems like you have more energy." Dockery also attributes having better balance to wearing his neuro-muscular mouth guard.[12]

The late founder of neuromuscular dentistry, Bernard Jankelson, coined the term when he and H.H. Dixon, a muscle physiologist at the University of Oregon School of Medicine, combined forces to relax the muscles of the jaw in order to find the optimal jaw position. According to his son, Robert Jankelson, who joined his father's practice in 1963, "What we hypothesized is if you can get the muscle healthy before you set the jaw position, you will have a much more desirable muscle to help you generate efficiency for either force or speed." Jankelson continues, "That mouthpiece... allows the best joint function and recruitment of the power muscles of the jaw; that's when you increase your athletic efficiency ... This power train goes all the way down, from the teeth, to the neck, the vertebrae, the back. The more you can get those articulations in a chain that will recruit the power muscles, that is your ultimate goal in repositioning the jaw."[13]

Of course, we believe that the muscles of the jaw relax the most when the airway is open, so performance is naturally enhanced by positioning the jaw for an open airway.

One additional factor for both health and athletic performance needs to be highlighted. At the Hindin Center, we also test our patients for heart rate variability (HRV), both before and after fitting dental appliances, to test whether or not the dental appliance is positioning the jaw for optimal results.

HRV is a measure of the inter-beat frequency of the heart rate, not just the change in speed of the heart rate, but the change in frequency of the beats on an on-going basis. HRV effectively

---

12 Falgoust, Michael J, "Neuromuscular Mouth Guard Draws Performance Debate," *USA Today* online, 11/17/2009. http://usatoday30.usatoday.com/sports/2009-11-16-neuromuscular-mouthguard-cover_N.htm
13 Ibid.

analyzes how well a person can deal with stress. Most importantly, HRV is a measure of a person's overall adaptability, and therefore their likelihood to survive.[14]

Since HRV indicates a person's ability to deal with stress as well as their ability to adapt physiologically to changing conditions, HRV also is an effective measure of potential peak athletic performance. One of the reasons that stretching before engaging in aerobic exercise is so important is that stretching can increase a person's HRV.[15]

We find that when we get a patient's jaw in the best Airway Centric® position, their HRV will improve. This demonstrates that the use of dental appliances to open a person's airway improves their overall health, including cardiovascular health, while also improving their athletic potential.

Actions for Improved Athletic Performance

» Get a night-time appliance to open your airway, custom-fitted by an Airway Centric® dentist, or get fitted for a CPAP machine by a physician or sleep specialist

» Get a daytime appliance, or mouth guard for athletes, custom-fitted not only to protect your teeth but also to open your airway for optimal daytime functioning

» Stretch! It will improve your heart rate variability, your health, your likelihood to survive, and your athletic abilities

» While you stretch, BREATHE, don't GASP!

---

14 Paraphrasing Dr Julian Thayer from his presentation, "Heart Rate Variability, Breathing and Pain," 2014 Conference of the American Academy of Physiological Medicine and Dentistry, Chicago, Illinois, "The Silent Airway Connection: Its Impact on Development, Performance & Health," April 25 and 26, 2014.

15 Mueck-Weymann, Michael, et al, "Stretching Increases Heart Rate Variability in Healthy Athletes Complaining about Limited Muscular Flexibility," *Clinical Autonomic Research,* February (2004) 14:15-18.

12

C H A P T E R

Integrating Airway Centric® Into Your Life

We are aware that this book gives you a great deal to digest. Congratulations for sticking with us to the very end! In this chapter we will summarize the take-home points about airway obstruction and its profound and long-term effects for children and adults. Our secondary purpose is to help you enlist your doctors, dentists, teachers, nutritionists and other healthcare professionals in the cause to increase awareness of the far-reaching effects of airway obstruction at all stages of life.

That's why we welcome you and even urge you to make copies of this chapter and give them to those who care for you and your children. It's unusual for authors to urge you to copy our material in today's world of copyright protections and lawsuits; however, it is important to us that every healthcare professional, every teaching professional and every parent becomes part of the Airway Centric® team, caring for children and adults who have airway issues yet may not even know it.

Like the blind men exploring the elephant, each part of the Airway Centric® team can contribute a piece of the puzzle until the entire picture becomes clear.

Many of us have never experienced the feeling of free and easy breathing. We hope we have raised your awareness of breathing freely as a bottom-line essential for good health and optimal performance.

What do you do with this awareness?

Become more informed. Share the information. And know that it is never too soon or too late to take action. You and your children, even your aging parents, will benefit from open airways and improved breathing.

The Airway Centric® Lifestyle

Airway obstruction, sleep-disordered breathing (SDB), obstructive sleep apnea (OSA), snoring, and other airway dysfunction such as mouth breathing affect us from cradle to grave. Silently and beneath the surface, the structure and function of your airway influences every aspect of your life, from birth and growth and development, to the early years and behavior and academic performance, on up to forgetfulness and fatigue in middle age, and early dementia in our elders. Open or obstructed airways affect sleep, inflammation levels, chronic disease, relationships, workplace performance and even how long we live and how we die. Given the far-reaching consequences of breathing disorders, it behooves all of us to do everything we can for our airways. Here's how to start now:

Questions to ask yourself and your loved ones:	Yes	Not Sure	No
Behavioral Questions:			
Are your sheets and blankets in a tangle when you wake up?			
Do you often awaken suddenly during the night without apparent reason?			
Do you have trouble waking up without caffeine?			
Do you often fall asleep in front of the TV or over a book in the evening, only to find you can't go back to sleep when you finally go to bed?			
Do you wake up to snack in the middle of the night?			

Questions to ask yourself and your loved ones:	Yes	Not Sure	No
Are you a mouth-breather? Are your lips apart when you sleep? (Ask someone to look)			
Daily Performance Questions:			
Do you often feel sleepy during the day?			
Do you have difficulty concentrating or remembering?			
Do you crave sugar and simple carbohydrates?			
Do you have difficulty losing weight?			
Do you experience sexual dysfunction (erectile dysfunction, lack of interest in sex)?			
Physiological Assessment Questions:			
Can you breathe easily through each nostril? (Press one closed and try)			
Do you have a narrow nose and face?			
Do your teeth seem crowded?			
Do you have scallops or ridges on your tongue?			
Do you have dark circles under your eyes?			
Is your tongue exceptionally large?			
Do you have large tonsils or adenoids?			
Can you put your tongue on the roof of mouth with your mouth wide open? (If not, you may have a tight frenum, which can cause airway problems)			
Do you have allergies that cause a stuffy nose?			
Health Issues Questions:			
Do you have health problems caused in part by chronic inflammation such as:			
Swollen joints/other swelling?			
Painful back?			
Arthritis?			
Type 2 Diabetes?			
Do you have Heart Disease?			
Do you have Arrhythmia?			
Do you have Alzheimer's Disease?			
Do you have Parkinson's Disease?			

If you answered "yes" to any of these questions, it could be a sign that you have airway-centered disorder, especially if any of your facial features match the descriptions given. If your neck size is also large, the chances increase greatly that you may have obstructive sleep apnea.

The Basics: What You Need to Know

What follows is a very brief summary of what you've learned in this book.

From Chapter 1 – Gasping for Life

» The central themes of this book constitute nothing less than a paradigm shift based on our 70 years of combined experience dealing with airway-centered disorders, and opening people's airways through dentistry as a practice of preventive medicine.

» Airway-centered disorders are the underlying, usually undetected causes of many conditions in both children and adults.

» We have epidemic levels of physical health issues, mental health issues, and diseases because we have an epidemic of obstructed airways.

From Chapter 2 – What Happened to Our Airways

» Before the advent of agriculture, human beings invariably had broad faces with widely-arched jaws, creating wide-open sinus passages as well as wide-open airways in the back of the mouth and throat (healthy airway patency).

» Darwinian Dentistry has revealed that, since the Industrial Revolution, soft diets and less breastfeeding have changed human faces from the ancestral pattern to a modern facial pattern. The modern face typically expresses an epigenetic dysfunction of long, narrow faces; a high, narrow palate; narrow jaws that do not provide enough space for either the teeth or the tongue; and correspondingly small sinus passages and blocked airways in the throat.

» The result of these facial changes has been an epidemic of airway-centered disorder, culminating in chronic issues of sleep-disordered breathing in people of all ages.

» These facial changes produced an increase in various SDB forms: mouth breathing, snoring, obstructive sleep apnea, hypopneas, and upper airway resistance syndrome.

From Chapter 3 – The Problems and the Airway Centric® Solution

» Our modern lifestyle—soft foods, less breastfeeding, ortho-dontic extraction of teeth, the use of head gear to correct overbites, and environmental exposure to toxins—has caused an epidemic of airway-centered disorders that have had disastrous effects on our national health.

» Without deep, restorative sleep, neither adults nor children can function well.

» ADHD rates have skyrocketed in recent decades: Between 1980 and 2007, ADHD increased by almost 700% in the United States.

» Today, nearly one-third of all children under 18 are overweight or obese, and 69.2% of adults are obese or overweight in the U.S.A.

» An open and functioning airway is the top priority in the well-being of the human organism. After all, if there is no breath, there is no life.

» The Goal of The Airway Centric® Approach: Focus on developing people's ability to breathe well while sleeping, in order to stop the epidemic of chronic diseases.

» While early treatment is always best (we have even treated newborns), ACD can be improved and often even reversed at any stage in life.

From Chapter 4 – Kids: Breathing, Learning, & Sleeping

» The National Sleep Foundation surveying parents found rates of sleep-disordered breathing in children as high as 18-19%.

» Frequent mouth breathing, snoring and sleep apnea in young children disrupt ideal brain development and produce changes in the prefrontal cortex that can have profound and far-reaching effects in terms of attention, behavior and learning abilities as well as anxiety and depression.

» Bed-wetting, nightmares, sleepwalking and colic are often associated with airway issues.

» Repeated bouts of tonsillitis are a signal that tonsils and adenoids should be removed immediately because they are impairing airflow, disrupting restorative sleep and negatively affecting brain development. The number one reason for removing tonsils today is obstruction not infection.

» This period of early childhood is critical in brain development, and sleep plays an important role in that development. A newborn's brain weighs only about 25% of an adult brain, but by age three, a child's brain is 80-85% the size of an adult's brain, and by age five, a child's brain is 90% the size of an adult's.

» Sleep-disordered breathing can damage the prefrontal cortex of children; some of these effects may be reversed with treatment, but some may be irreversible. Preventing sleep-disordered breathing in children is therefore imperative.

» Young children with SDBs may develop a "learning debt" that may "hamper subsequent school performance," and obstructive sleep apnea may lower a child's IQ by 10 points.

» Airway obstruction is linked to attention deficit and hyperactivity disorder (ADHD), learning disabilities, allergies, asthma and inflammatory disease.

» Children with the worst sleep problems are 40-60% more likely to have learning issues. SDB also increased the risk of behavioral difficulties by 40% at age 4 and 60% at age 7.

» By age 7, children with SDBs were 40-100% more likely to exhibit behavior problems that fit clinical diagnoses, according to researchers in the Avon Longitudinal Study.

» Early intervention is key—for both prevention and treatment. A child already diagnosed with ADHD at age 2 or 3 should have an evaluation of their sleep, ability to breathe through their nose, facial tone, jaw development, and the openness of their airway. This is particularly important in light of the fact that the Centers for Disease Control has found that 100,000 toddlers in the U.S. are being treated with ADHD medications like Ritalin and Adderall. Breastfeeding is important for creating an open nasal air passageway. In order to breastfeed, the child needs some nasal airway patency, including the absence of a tongue-tie.

» Orthodontists often erroneously remove teeth to provide room to produce straight teeth without spaces. This can result in recessed jaws and diminished airways. Do not allow an orthodontist to remove permanent teeth.

» Some airways are obstructed from the time of birth. Many premature infants have high narrow palates, making it difficult or impossible to breathe through the nose.

» Children who die of SIDS typically have a high, narrow palate, symptomatic of partially blocked airways. As the epiglottis begins to descend at ages 2-6 months, a child becomes more able to mouth-breathe, and if the sinuses are partially blocked, this may lead to mouth breathing, which in turn may increase the incidence of SDBs, possibly contributing to the occurrence of SIDS.

» If your child is a noisy sleeper, ask for a sleep screening to determine if there is SDB.

From Chapter 5 – Your Child's Face: Preventing Life-Long Problems

» A long narrow face is an indicator of an airway obstruction as the body struggles to breathe.

» Mouth breathing adversely changes the growth of the face. As a person adjusts to a stuffy nose by taking a life-giving breath more easily through the back up mechanism—the mouth—the face responds by growing longer, allotting more space to the mouth and less to the nasal passages.

» Children with airway obstructions typically have a retruded or receding lower jaw, a forward head posture, elongated face and a gummy smile. The forward and downward motion prompted by lack of nasal breathing and increased effort results in mouth breathing and often a bump on the nose.

» Nutrition also plays an important role in the shape of a child's face. Our modern diets, full of soft, processed foods, influence children's facial shape, how straight their teeth will be, as well as the openness of their airways.

» Consider a palate expansion if you see signs that a child has an airway obstruction. Palate expanders can be used as early as age 3. It is important that the correct appliance is utilized to achieve expansion in the needed directions.

» Intervene as early as possible. Do not wait to start palate expansion if there is narrowing of the airway or a high, vaulted arch of the upper palate.

From Chapter 6 – Sick and Tired of Feeling Sick and Tired

» Sleep-disordered breathing is a systemic condition, changing brain chemistry, the body's metabolism, hormone balance, and overall physical and mental wellbeing.

» Obstructive sleep apnea increases the likelihood of cardio-vascular disease, diabetes, obesity, acid reflux, and even fatal cancer.

» If you have diabetes, heart disease, arrhythmia, hypertension, osteoarthritis, back pain, hypothyroidism, chronic allergies or asthma, anxiety or depression, consider the possibility you have an airway obstruction.

» Metabolic syndrome refers to the body having an increased risk for an increasingly common triad of unhealthiness: obesity, diabetes, and cardiovascular disease. Treating sleep-disordered breathing is the number one overlooked method for reversing our nation-wide health decline.

» Opening the airway and easing breathing will almost always improve chronic health conditions, even for older adults.

» Poor sleep quality also triggers carbohydrate cravings by changing levels of leptin and grehlin in the brain, resulting in weight gain. Excess weight results in a vicious circle of more snoring and more sleep apnea in both adults and children.

» Chronic inflammation is also the result of chronic stress. Both are aggravated by poor sleep. Studies demonstrate that SDBs can elevate levels of inflammatory cytokines.

» Low energy even after seven or eight hours in bed is a sign of SDB. Do you complain often that you are exhausted? That's another sign of SDB and lack of restorative sleep.

» Insomnia, wakefulness in the middle of the night, snoring, restless legs, and tooth grinding are all signs of airway obstruction.

» Sleep apnea causes the body to go into a state of panic because breathing has stopped. Stress hormones are released and blood sugar drops, causing carbohydrate cravings.

» Disrupted sleep is an underlying cause of weight gain.

» Generalized inflammation associated with fragmented sleep causes the body to retain fat.

» Being overweight negatively affects sleep cycles and increases the risk of sleep apnea.

» Lack of restful sleep causes fatigue throughout the day, and we instinctively reach for sugar and simple carbohydrates to bring energy back up, only to have it crash again a couple of hours later.

» People who get six hours of sleep or less a night have a high risk of obesity.

» Clean up your sleep habits by choosing the right mattress; making your bedroom cool, comfortable and dark; banning television and other electronics from the bedroom; keeping a regular sleep schedule; getting regular exercise; and eating a healthy diet low in simple carbohydrates.

From Chapter 7 – Women and Sleep-Disordered Breathing

» Sleep-disordered breathing may present with a different set of symptoms in women than in men, typically including fatigue, morning headaches, and insomnia.

» Women more often suffer from upper airway resistance syndrome, which is subtler and therefore harder to detect. Not all sleep centers test for UARS.

» SDBs cause a stress response that activates the HPA Axis (hypothalamus-pituitary-adrenal), thus causing symptoms that mimic chronic fatigue and fibromyalgia, as well as anxiety disorders. Many women may experience such disorders without being tested for SDBs, especially UARS.

» Pregnancy is a crucial time for women to prevent SDBs, as women with SDBs are more likely to give birth prematurely, and SDBs have been shown to slow fetal heart rates.

» Menopause may lead to an increased risk of OSA in women, exacerbating health issues and promoting weight gain.

» There may be an increased risk of breast cancer from SDBs. In addition, sleep fragmentation has been shown to increase the risk of mortality from breast cancer.

From Chapter 8 – Mental Health and Blocked Airways

» Sleep-disordered breathing is associated with a variety of mental challenges: ADHD in children and adults, anxiety, depression, irritability, memory deficits, inability to concentrate, and decreased alertness.

» Imagine repeatedly being suffocated at night while you're trying to sleep. That's what people with sleep apnea deal with all night, every night. This leads to a physiological stress response, aka: anxiety.

» People with OSA wake up feeling lethargic, yet anxious. All day long, they are nervous and startle easily. Panic attacks set in over seemingly small issues. It is hard to think clearly. Anxiety becomes chronic and hard to manage.

» Research on veterans has found links between OSA and anxiety, and even stronger links between OSA and PTSD, suggesting there may be a bi-directional relationship between the two. Treating SDBs has been shown, when pursued over a course of months, to reduce symptoms of PTSD.

» Researchers at the New York University School of Medicine found an association between sleep-disordered breathing and biological brain changes that increase risk of Alzheimer's in thin, senior adults.

» Researchers have recently discovered what they call a "glymphatic system," which flushes toxins out of the brain while we sleep.

» 7. 50-80% of children with autism spectrum disorder experience sleep problems, compared to 9-50% of normally-developing children experiencing sleep problems. There may be a bi-directional relationship between SDBs and autism.

» Infants lying on their backs may be more susceptible to sleep-disordered breathing, and thus to a lack of healthy brain development. McCabe ties the "back to sleep" campaign, originating in 1992, with the high incidence of autism. While rates of SIDS deaths declined significantly due to this trend to have infants sleep on their backs, the rate of autism increased.

» The New York-based National Down Syndrome Society claims that 50-100% of individuals with Down syndrome have obstructive sleep apnea, and almost 60% of children with Down syndrome develop sleep problems by the age of 3.5 to 4 years.

» For people with Down syndrome, working with an OMT (orofacial myofunctional therapist) may be especially important to improve muscle tone as well as aid in the coordination of breathing and swallowing properly both night and day.

From Chapter 9 – Chronic Pain, Inflammation, and Your Airway

» A compromised airway will cause pain somewhere in the body.

» Pain causes stress, and stress causes inflammation, which causes more pain in a vicious cycle. SDB and OSA trigger both stress and inflammation and consequently, pain.

» If you treat the pain but ignore airway function—a rarely considered source of the problem—the pain simply moves to another place.

» If you have TMJ (temporomandibular joint dysfunction) or you have pain or clicking and popping sounds in your jaw, a slung-back jaw is a likely cause of your problem and your SDB.

» Many types of headache are linked to SDB.

» At least one-third of people with bruxism (teeth grinding) also have sleep-disordered breathing conditions, including sleep apnea and periodic leg movement. Headaches are also a common finding.

» Good posture and diaphragmatic breathing help open airways and relieve pain. In our practices, we have found that treating SDBs can eliminate many different types of pain: not only TMJ, but back, neck, shoulder, even pain in the hands as well as the pain of irritable bowel syndrome.

From Chapter 10 – Mental and Physical Daily Performance

» Your best performance at work, at play, and in the bedroom requires an open airway and a good night's sleep.

» People who work too much don't get enough sleep. And people who don't sleep well enough have slowed cognitive function. Reducing nighttime sleep by as little as 1.5 hours for just one night could mean a 32% drop in daytime alertness.

» According to the Centers for Disease Control, "Driving while drowsy causes an estimated 1,550 fatalities annually, as well as 40,000 non-fatal injuries each year in the United States."

» Sleep deprivation and OSA have caused some of the major accidents and disasters of recent decades, including the Chernobyl meltdown, the grounding of the Exxon Valdez, the Three-Mile Island Disaster, the train wreck in New York in 2013, and the explosion in Bhopal, India, chemical plant.

» Researchers in Switzerland found that workers with sleep problems were 62% more likely to experience workplace injuries.

» Workers with OSA were almost 14 times more likely to have had job-performance problems, according to a study, including sleeping on the job or missing a day's work, during just a four-week period. People with OSA and excessive daytime sleepiness were almost four times as likely to have had a pay cut or miss a promotion.

» There's an established association between sleep apnea and sexual performance. Treatment of OSA leading to a good night's sleep can improve and preserve sexual function in men and even reverse erectile dysfunction.

» In women, a study out of Sweden showed women with OSA had significantly more sexual dysfunction than woman without it.

From Chapter 11 – Airways and Athletic Performance

» Adequate sleep is essential to athletic performance, and adding just an hour or two of sleep per day can dramatically improve results on the basketball or tennis court, running track, and elsewhere.

» Since HRV (heart rate variability) indicates a person's ability to deal with stress, as well as their ability to adapt physiologically to changing conditions, HRV also represents an effective measure of potential peak athletic performance.

» When Michael Jordan stuck out his tongue to make winning shots time-after-time in the last seconds of games, he was intuitively placing his jaw in the Airway Centric® appliance position; this allowed him to enter "the zone."

» When athletes use AirwayCentric® oral appliances to optimize jaw position to open their airways, we see improvements in posture, balance and performance

» A double-blind study with football players used a MORA, or mandibular orthopedic repositioning appliance, which repositions the jaw in a forward position to open the airway. In this study, the MORA reduced the number and severity of injuries, especially knee injuries, while also increasing strength.

» One measure of potential athletic performance is heart rate variability (HRV). HRV is also a measure of good health, and only an open airway and absence of SDBs can maintain a good HRV.

» HRV measurements are used to determine the accuracy of the fit of an appliance. The greater the improvement in HRV, the better the fit of the appliance, and the greater the potential for peak athletic performance.

What You Can Do

If you suspect that an airway obstruction may underlie your health issues or those of your spouse or child, here's how to take action:

» **Action: Be an Informed Consumer.** Be an advocate for yourself, your spouse and your child. Ask your doctor, dentist and/or ENT specialist for an airway evaluation. If any of them identify an airway impairment, ask for a sleep study. If the study is for a child, ask for a referral to a board-certified pediatric sleep specialist.

Sadly, many doctors, dentists and healthcare professionals are not aware of the vital importance of an unobstructed airway for all aspects of health. So, you can add an educator's hat on top of your advocate's hat.

» **Action: Be persistent.** We've developed the Airway Centric® educational model for lifelong health precisely because so many medical professionals are not trained in or overlook the importance of clear airways and restorative sleep to the entire human organism. Your persistence could help put the airway at the center of medical awareness and diagnosis and educate healthcare professionals, parents and teachers to evaluate for airway obstruction.

» **Action: Do-It-Yourself.** The following are a few do-it-yourself techniques you can use today. They are not cures, and they will most likely still lead you to professional help, but they will be an indicator if SDB is a factor in your health problems. None of the following is intended to diagnose or cure any disease. We recommend that you consult with your physician about any health issues you are currently experiencing.

- *Nasal breathing aids:* You can purchase Breath Right strips that are placed on the outside of your nose or Mute products that fit inside the opening of the nose. These devices may reduce nasal congestion, open the nasal passages and reduce snoring. If you experience a noticeable improvement in your daytime energy after using these for a few days, you may have SDB. If so, obtain a comprehensive exam by seeing your doctor, a sleep specialist, and an Airway Centric® dentist.

- *Nasal spray:* We prefer Xlear, a natural combination of xylitol and saline solution that helps moisturize the sinus and nasal passages. It also works by disrupting the biofilm and eliminating hiding spots for bacteria. It doesn't contain drying antihistamines and decongestants and may help with nighttime breathing, particularly if you are mouth breathing or snoring because of allergies or sinusitis.

- *Sleep on your side:* This is the best position for an open airway as long as you are not curled tight in a fetal position.

- *Have the right pillow:* Your pillow should not raise your head; it should just support it at a straight angle. Get a firm pillow and change your pillow often, especially if allergies are a component of your airway obstruction. Consider a foam wedge that elevates your head and upper body; you insert this under your bottom sheet on top of your mattress.

- *Diaphragmatic or yoga breathing:* Consciously deepening your breathing can help expand your lungs, oxygenate your entire system and de-stress your body.

- *Lose weight:* Excess weight is definitely a factor in SDB and OSA. Losing weight will help break the particularly insidious vicious cycle of fragmented sleep: SDB-stress-inflammation-fatigue-carbohydrate cravings.

- *Watch your partner:* He or she may have no idea if SDB is taking place, but you will.

All of these DIY strategies can help if you have a mild airway obstruction. But there is no way you can know what is happening when you are sleeping. Your partner might tell you, but you might or might not believe reports of snoring, snorting, gasping and more. However, you do know all-too-well when you're not sleeping and you're exhausted.

We'll warn you here: If you have a serious SDB or OSA problem, the strips, nasal spray, even the foam wedge will almost immediately help you feel much better rested and less fatigued. However, they haven't addressed the underlying problem, which can be life threatening. Please get a professional evaluation so you can truly rest easy.

» **Action: If you are pregnant or planning a pregnancy: Get prenatal nutrition counseling.** If you have any indication that you have SDB, include an airway/sleep screening as part of your prenatal to identify snoring and OSA. Sleep apnea during the second and third trimesters of pregnancy can affect your baby's epigenetics and affect the airway at birth.

Ask your OBGYN, midwife or doula to assess your baby's naso-maxillary complex, airway function, high dental arch and frenum at birth. Be sure they know what to look for. Your airway problem and your body's response to it can have serious consequences for your baby.

Ask your lactation counselor for an evaluation of your baby's suck-swallow-breathe reflex (especially important for preemies) and their ability to latch onto the breast, keeping the airway open. Be certain the baby is nasal breathing, not mouth breathing.

If there are any signs of an airway problem, consider having a craniosacral adjustment. Sometimes during the birth process, the soft cranial bones do not move properly. We've seen this simple adjustment change a baby's entire personality: the baby becomes calmer, cries less and looks healthier. This adjustment encourages nursing and latching-on in babies who have been reluctant.

» **Action: Observe your children: Be aware of mouth breathing.** Watch your child's tongue for telltale ridges associated with mouth breathing, and look out for forward slouching posture.

» **Action: Listen for noisy sleeping, even at a very early age.** This can be snoring, gasping, groaning or coughing. Behavioral concentration and learning problems are potential signs of airway obstruction.

It's never too late to address the problem, but it's important to do what you can as early as possible for children. Because children's brain development takes place so rapidly in the early years, airway obstruction can hinder that development and have consequences that will continue throughout the child's life.

» **Action: Contact an Airway Centered Practitioner.** Airway problems can be difficult to recognize and only get worse with time. If observations of yourself and your family indicate that a problem exists, seek professional help and the right help. All practitioners are cognizant of these issues and their importance.

What we and the Airway Centric® model can do for you: If there is any indication of SDB or OSA in your life, your partner's or your child's, please get an airway evaluation from a qualified professional.

How to Find Help

85% of practitioners will not be aware of the "hidden airway" paradigm, which explains why 85% of the population of airway, sleep and breathing disordered patients are still unrecognized and undiagnosed.

At birth find a midwife, doula or lactation consultant who can help with breastfeeding if you or your baby are having difficulty. There is a group called the IATP, which is the International Affiliation of Tongue Tied Professionals. If a tethered tongue is the issue, they should be able to help or see Tongue Tie Babies Support Group on Facebook or your local pediatric ENT trained in airway and sleep.

Some premature infants are born as mouth breathers and may be unable to obligately nasal breathe during breastfeeding. Consult an occupational therapist (OT) or a myofunctional therapist (MFT).

Children with low tone in their tongue, throat and facial muscles are also best addressed by OTs and MFTs. Myofunctional therapists can be found at:

AOMT: www.aomtinfo.org

IAOM: www.iaom.com

Mouthbreathing, snoring and apnea are not normal in children. Noisy breathing is not a sign that a child is sleeping soundly. The Pediatric Sleep Questionnaire is a good starting point for parents and professionals who are trying to determine if there is a problem.

Some pediatric ENTs have specialty training in airway, breathing and sleep disorders. In NYC, Westchester and Rockland Counties, we are lucky to have some excellent physicians who understand the relationship between small airways, large tonsils and adenoids and neurobehavioral and neurocognitive disorders. Some ENTs and ENT / plastic surgeons can support the nasal airway so it does not collapse with increased airflow.

To locate an Airway Centered Practitioner go to the "Find a Dr" section on www.foundationforairwayhealth.org and www.AAPMD. org.

Remember the 80/20 rule. Until now, only 20% of the practitioners you see will be able to recognize an airway/sleep/breathing problem.

There is a growing interest in Airway Centric® orthodontics. The foundationforairwayhealth.org website lists non retractive AC orthodontic organizations and individuals who can help you, your child, grandchild, or loved one.

Beware of the orthodontist who tells you that your child's mouth is too small and that permanent teeth need to be extracted. Yes, our mouths are getting smaller due to epigenetic factors; however, jaws can be expanded at a young age in a matter of months and our colleagues like Bill Hang, John and Michael Mew, Duane Grummons, Kevin Boyd, David Singh, Darick Nordstrom, James Bronson, Brian Hockel, Darick Nordstrom, Jim Bronson, Barry Raphael, Derek Mahoney, Brock Rondeau, Steve Galella, David Buck and others are doing it and teaching it every day. Look for an airway-centered, Airway Centric® airway-friendly orthodontist or general dentist in your area who values the airway and builds the most beautiful, healthiest face around an open airway.

Invisalign – Most orthodontists and general dentists trained in Invisalign have historically focused on straightening teeth. Airway Centered dentists are using Invisalign to expand the dental arch with the emphasis on establishing an airway, secondarily supporting the temporomandibular joints, and finally aligning teeth.

The earlier the intervention orthodontically to expand the palate and develop the airway, the greater the positive impact on the developing brain.

We are forming pods around the country that include an AC Dentist, orthodontist, pediatric dentist, SLP, Myofunctional Therapist, physical therapist, sleep specialist, ENT, pediatric ENT, oral surgeon and pulmonologist.

Physical therapists who have been trained by Mariano Rocabado P.T. from Santiago, Chile or Gregg Johnson from IPA (www.InstituteofPhysicalArt.com) are recommended.

Many sleep physicians routinely prescribe CPAP, even for mild OSA, to the exclusion of other therapies. Mild and moderate apnea may be treated successfully with oral appliance therapy. Moderate and severe OSA with associated comorbidities such as cardiovascular disease may be best served with CPAP.

It's never too late to intervene. If you or a loved one is losing their memory, lack of oxygen and disturbed sleep may be a contributing factor. Consider: Sharp Again Naturally www.sharpagain.org

If you are seeking help, visit www.AAPMD.org or www.foundationforairwayhealth.org to find a practitioner for you or your loved ones.

Oral Appliances

There are palatal expanders for young children as young as 3 years of age. Some are removable and others are cemented in or fixed in place. The hard part is finding an orthodontist who is willing to do this early phase 1 treatment.

For those children who still need orthodontics at age 7 or 8, there is BioBloc Orthotropics popularized by specialists Dr John Mew and Dr William M. Hang. This technique maximizes the airway space and provides the largest airway and most beautiful faces.

For headache patients, Dr Michael Gelb uses a modification of the original Gelb appliance or MORA (mandibular orthopedic repositioning appliance) during the day, and usually a Farrar upper anti-retrusion appliance at night. For more serious SDB cases, we use a variety of appliances including the Oasys, Somnomed, SUAD, TAP, Herbst, Snor no More, Respire, EMA, Silencer as well as hybrid designs with CPAP.

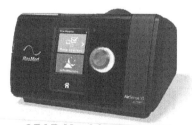

CPAP Machine

Currently we are recommending a milled appliance from Prosomnus called $MicrO_2$ which does not impinge upon the tongue. 3D printed appliances are also very effective and includes the Panthera as well as the Narval from ResMed.

CPAP Machine: Continuous Positive Airway Pressure machine, this device is a pump that consists of a tight-fitting mask over the face or nose or nasal prongs that increases pressure in the airway so it does not collapse during sleep. This is a very effective means of addressing SDB and OSA. However, many patients can't tolerate the machine. It can be noisy and uncomfortable. If your airway obstruction is severe apnea, a CPAP machine will be recommended for you. Your life may depend on being able to use it every night. Sometimes a combination of a CPAP machine and oral appliance will provide the best workable solution. Your dentist, ENT or sleep specialist can help you make adjustments to increase your comfort.

Nutritional and airway problems are often found together. One can lead to the other; each can make the other worse. It can be a "perfect storm" leading to a myriad of health and performance problems. Optimal treatment requires a collaborative treatment approach.

You, your spouse and your children cannot have a healthy, happy and productive life with a poorly structured and improperly functioning airway. If you are reading this book, of course you are breathing, but with what effort and at what price? The cost can affect every part of your body, your brain, your performance and your relationships.

We hope *GASP* will reveal whether you have an unrecognized airway problem. Remember: 85% of the population of airway, sleep and breathing disordered patients are still unrecognized and undiagnosed. Get screened. Get diagnosed. Get optimal treatment.

Let *GASP* be the guide for your new beginning of hope, improved health and performance. Share *GASP* with your family and friends. Be part of the Airway Health Paradigm.

Index

Index

Index

Made in the USA
San Bernardino, CA
18 March 2017